TANTRIC & KASHMIRI

MASSAGES

. Six illustrated protocols step–by–step
. Tips and techniques for beginners

MICHÈLE LARUE

AVERTISSEMENT

About the author

Since 1996, Michèle Larue has published many erotic short stories in French and in English. Her publications in French include a series of sex manuals, such as *Osez booster votre libido* («Dare Boosting Your Libido») and *Osez le Sexe Tantrique* («Have a go at Tantric Sex»), all published by Éditions la Musardine. She has investigated all the different ways we can develop and refine our sensuality. Today the niceties of Tantric and Kashmiri massage are her field of predilection, as detailed in her latest manual in French, *L'Art du massage tantrique et cachemirien*.

Illustrations © Axterdam

Translation: Noël Burch

Layout: designed by Nathalie Amae

Book cover: designed by Jean-Marc Eldin

Cover photograph: Stock Adobe

Tantric & Kashmiri Massages © 2018 – by MICHÈLE LARUE

43 FIGURES ILLUSTRATE THE MOUVEMENTS AND POSITIONS OF EACH TYPE OF MASSAGE

INTRODUCTION

As I received various Tantric massages in the course of my research, I tried to conceptualize the different techniques used and the impulse which gives birth to voluptuousness and transmits love, the joy of sharing emotions and sensations through the most powerful of all forms of contact, the sense of touch.

This led directly to my taking note of what the different Tantric and Kashmiri massages have in common and where the difficulties lie. Of course, there are as many different massages as there are masseurs and masseuses and yet the same sequences of positions and moves recurred regularly during these exchanges. The protocols and practices described in this manual will provide a preliminary framework for the moves to be performed and transitions to be smoothed out, as well as tips and tricks meant to increase the fluidity of a Tantric massage. Readers may simply draw their initial inspiration from these and go on to massage freely with the open heart advocated by all Tantrism.

The manual also offers solo exercises which will put you more in touch with yourself and with others: breathing techniques, self-massages, Yoga positions specifically related to the opening of your hearts for both partners. I shall also set forth some rules that it is important to know, even if they are forgotten once they have become second nature.

PLAYING THE ORGAN

Because of their all-inclusive nature — the fact that they include the genitals— the full body massages associated with the Tantra are termed "holistic". They awaken feelings of voluptuousness thanks to the sexual energy released at its source, around the genitals and at the bottom of the sacrum, diffusing it throughout the body. Despite what many think, they are not "sexual massages" —unless they are specifically designated as such. The word "Tantric" is often misunderstood. Pictures of bare-breasted masseuses promising "naturist", i.e. sexual Tantric massages abound on the net. An authentic Tantric or Kashmiri massage involves sensuality, emotion and spirituality, but its goal is neither an orgasm nor ejaculation, which are only brief moments of pleasure compared with an hour and a half of sensuousness. Some professionals have grown weary of this confusion and prefer to call them "energetic" or "meditative" massages.

Osho (1931-1990) the charismatic popularizer of the Tantra, advised the active partner in a massage to "play the organ" lovingly, using the power of touch to develop mutual harmony. The energy exchanged through a loving touch brings happiness to the giver whose hands are charged with compassion. The receiver enters into a state of sensual meditation and becomes a musical instrument whose sensibility vibrates to the loving touch, connected with emotions to which we are no longer accustomed. The opening of the heart enables both partners to intensify the concert of feminine values which are the bases of the Tantra and the fundamentals of care ethics.

SELF-HELP

Today, the prominence of personal development and the ethics of care —especially through massage— may be regarded as a therapeutic response to the rampant violence in urban life in our time. Assailed as we are by stimuli and enticements of every sort, rediscovering our bodies, communing with our sensibility and that of our partners, even restoring a relationship to the sacred through shamanism or the Tantra can strengthen our sense of rootedness weakened by stress. Is the prediction wrongly attributed to the great French novelist André Malraux, "the twenty-first century will be spiritual or will not be", turning out to be accurate?

CHAPTER 1

GENEALOGY OF TANTRIC MASSAGE

The most ancient Tantric scriptures are known no less than 5,500 years old in their oral form but were not written down until the 7th century of our era. These sacred writings are called Tantras (weaving the cloth) and are in the form of a dialogue between the god Shiva, the representation par excellence of male energy, and the goddess Shakti, the dynamic female energy which ensures the vibrations of the universe. Shakti, often represented as a yoni (vulva), is the serpent goddess sleeping coiled at the base of the sacrum where the sacred fire burns. She must be united with the god Shiva at the tip of the cranium, the creative source of sleep, often represented as a lingam (phallus). It integrates desire and spirituality through the regular practice of exercises and rituals, transforming sexual desire into such positive dispositions as compassion. According to a Tantric text: "What a male Tantrika achieves in a year, a female devotee obtains in a single day."

Tantric Shivaism, a branch of Hinduism, has its roots in the ancient Dravidian worship of the Great Goddess. Among the Dravidian peoples, whose civilization spread westward from what is now Pakistan to the Mediterranean and south to Sri Lanka, woman embodied spontaneity and openness, as she would later among the Celts. She represented harmonious strength, bravery and depth of vision, the love of nature and respect for it.

The Aryans, the Muslims from the Middle East and the puritanical English, all the subsequent civilizations in India, imposed their traditional moral order, the inferiorization of women, monogamy and varying degrees of prudery. Forced to go underground at the end of the 10th century, Tantrism was no doubt kept alive in tiny communities scattered across the different countries where they had settled.

THE NEW AGE ERA

In the 1970s, Rajneesh Chandra Mohan Jain, aka Osho, an Indian Guru ("spiritual master" in Sanskrit), revamped the ancient scriptures and invented the precepts of Tantric massage on the basis of the essential components of the Tantra. His ashram at Pune in northern India was attended by thousands of young people who suffered from a lack of physical contact and emotion and who were attracted by the sexual freedom that prevailed there. The Tantra was freely interpreted in a context of merry promiscuity. Nowadays with the tourist trade, it is almost impossible to find an authentic Tantric massage in India, even supposing that there actually still exist honest practitioners who are not simply exploiting the fashion for massages and the "democratization" of the Tantra.

Like Buddhism, Tantrism spread to the West with the New Age movement in the eighties. Westerners trained in these techniques in the United States and later in Europe. Two women, both Tantra leaders, published books describing their practices and what they experienced. They still organize workshops and internships based on the teachings of Osho. Margo Anand has settled in Bali and teaches a set of practices meant to achieve ecstasy called Sky Dancing. The Canadian Ma Premo lives in close proximity with Amerindians.

During the nineties, a certain contempt for feminine values caused a cult of the exploit to take precedence over sensibility and the virtues of the heart. Nurses in day-care centers no longer touched the babies for fear of being accused of sexual abuse. After years of life together, many couples neglected the pleasures of touching one another. In 2001, the terrorist attack on the twin towers in New York generated a feeling of helplessness and called into question many of our certainties. People withdraw into themselves. Yoga, meditation, Shiva's dancing and Tantric massages attracted again Western youths who turned to self-help techniques and care ethics, devoting themselves to the intensification of their feelings and the protection of their health in order to make the most of their lives.

CHAPTER 2

THE TANTRIC VISION OF THE BODY

A Tantric vision of life and of oneself is essential for the person giving the massage. The receiver may very well know nothing of Tantra, in which case a first massage constitutes an initiation that may open the way to self-discovery, to being be in tune with ourselves thanks to a recovered sense of spontaneity, sensuality and the vibrations of our emotions.

The Tantric vision primarily involves improving our capacity for listening to ourselves. We develop mindfulness while opening our hearts and sharing, two attitudes in life which are not always easy to combine: self-awareness can eventually degenerate into narcissism or egotism. Thus, the willingness to share must take priority.

REDISCOVERING SENSUALITY

Lying naked, being touched all over our body allows us to rediscover the innocence that was ours before puberty, the innocence of childhood and the happy days spent exploring our sense of touch. We feel alive! "The Tantra is a relaxation in the present, we are a blank page, we rediscover our senses like a child", says the Tantric Canadian leader Ma Premo. And this new feeling of innocence is certainly superior to the first since it is consciously desired. Some people have not been touched in this way since their first baths, when their mother washed them. In the practice, while you are bonded with your partner by an increasingly spontaneous link, both of you will feel unified within yourselves and connected with the universe. In the silence of those moments, the giver and the receiver of the massage find a harmony with themselves, an ecstatic peace through this bodily contact via the skin.

SHEDDING THE "ARMOR"

Since it targets our sensibility and our spirituality, this type of massage helps us rid ourselves of our "coat of armour", those useless layers that conceal from us the person we really are. It can bring forth feelings from our deepest self. Some people open up right away, others require time to let go of everything that weighs them down.

THE FOUR BODIES

A Tantric massage targets several senses at once: our sense of touch, naturally, but also our eyesight via a beautiful decorative scheme, while our sense of smell is bewitched by the fragrances from a dispenser or the massage oil, while our sense of hearing is charmed by soft music. The massage addresses the four bodies:

- The mental body
- The physical body
- The emotional body
- The spiritual body

PLUNGING INTO OURSELVES

Indeed, the Tantra invites us to turn inwards, to take —or retake— possession of our body without the intervention of the mind, rediscovering forgotten sensations. This immersion in our consciousness may also be achieved through a serious practice of meditation and Yoga. Consciousness —our state of being between two thoughts, "the consciousness of all things" as Abhinavagupta, the grand master of the Kashmiri Tantra, phrased it in the 10th century. In this metaphysics, consciousness, whose presence we can sense within ourselves when the chatterbox of our thoughts has fallen silent, is "the origin of all beings underpinning the universe," in the words of the *Baghavad Gitâ*. Our breath is the bearer of our spiritual being as well as the nutriment of our chakras. Caring for oneself and knowing oneself while celebrating the radiant omnipresence which each of us carries within constitutes the basis of this spirituality.

ATTENTION WITHOUT INTENTION

If we pay less attention to the present, it is because we find it rather uninteresting. We have a thousand things we plan to do in the future and we find our day to day routine dull, we'd rather project ourselves into the future hoping to experience something different or else we spend our time mulling over the past. We often live off-balance, straining towards the future when at bottom, there is nothing but the present moment, experienced through the true joy which sparkles inside us. Tantric massage is a sensual experience close to the state of meditation: you are here and now, in an eternal present. The receiver is content with merely existing. As for the giver, they are in a state of pure attentiveness yet the giver's hands convey no intention, not even that of doing good to their partner. This is difficult for beginners who want to do the right thing, who tend to put too much effort into the massage so keen are they on doing the other person good. Benevolent detachment will come with practice.

Topspace and subspace

The massage's giver benefits as much as the receiver through the same medium: skin-contact. However, they are in two different states since the one is active and the other passive. Their mental spaces resemble the "topspace" and "subspace" to which practitioners of bondage (shibari) refer. The topspace is the extremely focused space of control inhabited by the giver. The benefits they derive from this moment reside in the mastery and refinement of their moves vis-a-vis their partner, the gift, the honing of their attentiveness. Their pleasure is very similar to that of the shibari "ripper", tying up their model with ropes. The receiver inhabits the subspace. They are passive and gradually relax thanks to an absolute confidence in the giver. Their letting-go, the abandonment of any subjectivity, activates the secretion of endorphins: they enter into a state of pleasant floating and come out of this shared moment liberated and enriched.

SPANDA: VIBRATION AND SPACE

In Sanskrit, spand means vibration, pulsation. In the Kashmiri Tantra, "the vibration of the One" is at the origin of the evolution of space and the universe. According to that philosophy, the organism of each human being is part of a larger and unique whole, and possesses its own rhythms and vibration as do the planets and nature itself. The energy in our body is perpetually in motion just like the universe. The vibrations in each of its cells generate the bioelectric currents that run through it. Our emotions give rise to some vibrations and cause others to change. The human body is thus considered to be an energy phenomenon. "At one end of the spectrum, at the physical level, this energy is expressed in sexual activity. At the other end, at the level of the nervous system and the brain, the energy is perceived as ecstasy," (Margo Anand, *The Art of Sexual Ecstasy*). In the Tantra, we pay special attention to our perceptions, our sensations and our emotions. A feeling of full awareness brings with it a sense of freedom which is quite different from that achieved in the days of the New Age movement, those happy-go-lucky days when hedonism, desire and spontaneity were all the rage.

HARMONIZING THE YIN AND THE YANG

The Tantric vision is to be found in Taoist thought and in the ancient practices associated with it. In both China and India today, dualism is still seen as complementary: the yin and the yang are the two parts of a single whole, whereas Western philosophy tends to separate and divide. The world's harmony is maintained thanks to the balance between these two constantly changing forces. This cosmic unity in the Tao —the Way, the All— appears to us as male/female but also in such complimentary oppositions as hot/cold, full/empty, night/day, sun/moon.

The yin is female and is associated with the moon, the earth, spring-water and rain, rest and emptiness, the young girl, the tiger and the turtle. The yang is male and is associated with the sun, the sky, clouds, fire, fullness, action, dragons. The yang is also wild, violent desire, virile strength and the warrior's derring-do. But we must remember that in every yang person lies some yin as well and vice versa. For the yang man, opening up to yin means letting in the Other without losing his own specific properties.

Tantric massages and cradling sessions in warm water (see watsu at the beginning of **Chapter 19**) are aimed at harmonizing the yin and the yang within us, the female and male, calming our mental agitation, replacing it by a powerful connection with the total consciousness. In a Tantric massage, the yang touch is the firmer and is more frequently used than the yin touch which tends to bring our sensibility to the surface of the skin (see **yin and yang** touches in **Chapter 6**).

Men and emotions

Men are generally not interested in certain parts of their bodies, which their sensibility is programmed to neglect. Thus as the massage makes him aware of it bit by bit, a man will gradually recover his body. Some men who have an autonomy deficit sometimes fall prey to contradictions they have not tried to resolve or were unable to do so. A man lacking in yin will find that a Tantric massage strengthens it in him. He will discover the strength of his emotions, often considered to be the sole province of women in our patriarchal societies. One often hears of men bursting into tears at the end of a good Tantric massage.

SEX AS A SOURCE OF ENERGY

The area of the sacrum contains a supply of vital energy —also called sexual energy. Tantric techniques (orbital breathing, Tantric stimulation, massage, etc.) release this energy and allow it to nourish our whole body. How can we neglect such a treasure? For many of us, sexuality is more real than the soul, all the more so as it contains our entire personal history. "Indeed, it is through sex, that imaginary point determined by our sexual arrangements, that each of us must pass in order to grasp our own intelligibility." (Michel Foucault, *History of Sexuality*). Through the work we do on ourselves, through our attention to our bodies, we discover the truth of our being in our sexual desires.

One of the 22 schools of Yoga, Kundalinî Yoga, taught in California in the heydays of the hippy movement by yogi Bajan, the inventor of Yogi Tea, spread through all the big cities. Its postures, breathing techniques and mantras make it possible to relate to one's feelings and awaken the much-vaunted "Kundalinî". This is that immense store of energy "coiled" at the bottom of the sacrum. Yoga also enables the practitioners to keep their pelvic region loosened up through certain exercises described below.

The Kundalinî

In Yoga and the Tantra, the Kundalinî is a powerful form of energy located at the bottom of the spinal column. In Tantric iconography it is symbolized by a coiled snake and associated with the Indian goddess Shakti. One of the goals of the breathing techniques and meditation is to awaken the Kundalinî whose ascension will integrate the seven chakras and facilitate our spiritual awakening (Samaras) and a high degree of self-awareness.

THE BODY IN MOTION

THE TANDAVA DANCE

In the sixties and seventies, the hippies danced to Indian music, swinging their arms with a long colored scarf dangling from their fingertips. Nowadays, that free-style dancing is to be found in Tantra workshops under the name of Tandava or Shiva's dance. It is meditation in motion. Compared with Taichi and its long and difficult to learn sequences, the absence of any choreography makes the movements purely intuitive.

- Your body starts moving to a rhythmical or leisurely music.
- Breathe deeply.
- Loosen up your pelvis, your shoulders, your arms and your neck.
- Follow your own rhythm and move any way you feel, rediscover spontaneity.
- You can alternate slow movements with more agitated phases: this "cosmic dance" is meant to represent the cycles of the universe, including the chaotic phases of its successive evolutions.

Dancing regularly at home puts us in a good mood and dispels the tiny tensions in our body. In a Tantra workshop, the dancing can last as long as 30 minutes, plenty of time for letting go. This duration favours the secretion of endorphins, the hormones favoring a gentle sense of well-being.

SHAKING

With music or without, shake your body from head to foot as in an animist trance or a rumba. For 15 minutes we become our body and nothing else. Agitating the body empties the head. The shaking may be followed by the previous exercise, provided we take a pause between the two: a few moments of calm between two jouncings of the body, lying flat on the floor and allowing what you have just experienced to float inside you, your feelings, the music that carried you away. Shaking dissolves the knots blocking our emotions and keeping our awareness under wraps. Derived from tribal trances and their effects, the technique was invented in Osho's ashram. Some animist societies still use it in their ritual trances.

Chapter 3

OPENING YOUR HEART

The Tantra pays special attention to the heart, designated as the seat of absolute love, of the divine and of the Self. The chakra which resonates throughout our body is the heart (see **Chapter 5**). The heart is that hypersensitive vital organ which breaks down in the event of stress or an emotional shock. It can even give up on us altogether when the shock is too violent. When our emotions dwell on the same old things, they affect the other main organs as well, the much talked-about second brain, located in the intestines and the stomach. Even our lungs react by contracting when we are unhappy. Giving or receiving a massage brings us to open our heart, develops our capacity to relate to others and to the world. The exercises described below help to open your heart and develop your positive energy.

THE INNER SMILE

Print the smile on your face and inject it into your heart to enrich the moments of sharing and make yourself more receptive. Practice makes perfect, a smile deliberately displayed can alter your mood for the better and ultimately delight you. Learn to smile by cultivating your vital energy. Our smile develops our necessary love for others but also our love for ourselves. Print it

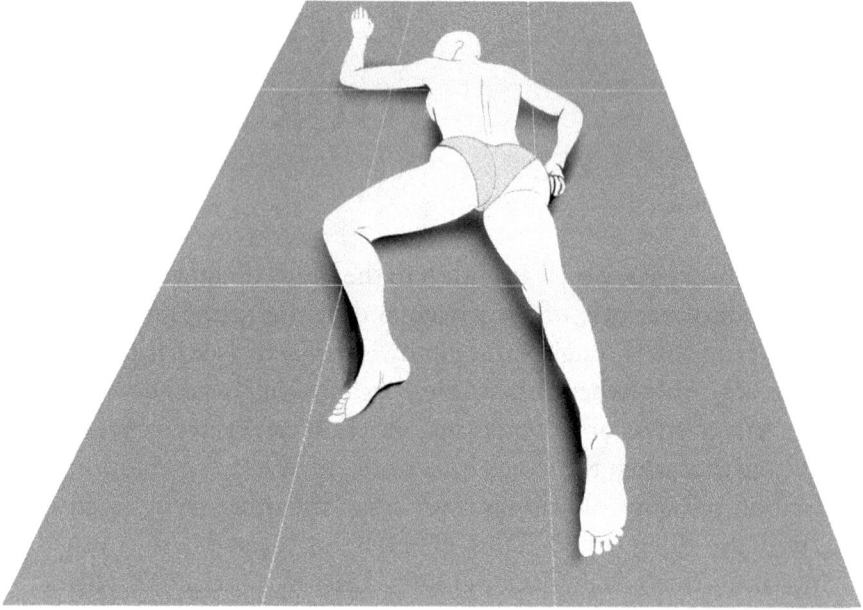

The Svastika posture releases the heart from the various tensions around it. The position awakens our sensations and emotions and enables you to open up to others.

1. The Svastika Posture

TANTRIC AND KASHMIRI MASSAGES

on your face and it will bathe your heart. This may be more difficult for a man brought up to behave in a manly way, than it is for
a woman. Like compassion, kindness and gentleness, a smile is
still associated with submissiveness in certain societies.

A YOGA POSTURE: THE SVASTIKA

This Yoga posture is the oldest of all: it goes back 5,000 years!
Long before it was appropriated by the Nazis, it was the cosmic
symbol for perpetual motion around a fixed point: the wheel
turns in the right direction, propitious for good health and luck.
In China, the corresponding ideogram means eternity or the
heart of Buddha. The Svastika posture releases the heart from the
various tensions around it. The position awakens our sensations
and emotions and enables you to open up to others.

- Lying flat on your stomach, head turned to the left, arms in
  candlestick position: slide your left knee towards your left
  elbow and bend your right arm in the opposite position to
  your left. Your left arm is bent at a 90° degree angle, forearm
  uppermost. Your right arm is similarly bent with the hand
  pointing down. Your elbows are lined up.
- Breathe quietly through the nose focusing your attention on
  the area of your heart.
- Hold the pose for 10 minutes.
- Come out of it by lowering the left knee and then the left
  arm.
  Turn over slowly on your back.
Let the effect of this position, also known as Baby Krishna, "brew"
inside you by relaxing with arms and legs outstretched in an X to
maximize the effect of the position. Your heart will be brimming
with love for yourself and for those around you, smiling, receptive and full of good will. figure 1).

MASSAGING ONE'S OWN THYMUS AND BREASTS

1. THE THYMUS

Sitting cross-legged, the skin of your buttocks stretched back to expose your anus and sacrum, breathe in while pulling your shoulders back and down. Next, throwing your head back, contract your pubococcygeus muscle, between the sex and the anus. Now breathe out, relaxing the anus and the perineum and bowing your head slightly. In this way, you can tone up thymus, an important gland for the secretion of hormones that make you feel good, located at the top of the thorax.

2. THE BREASTS

Describe little inward circles with both hands on your breasts, breathing deeply through your nose. Massaging your own breasts draws your internal energy to an area which is seldom addressed. Asians say that Western sensuality is confined to the lower body and disregards the upper parts.

Women, but also men, whose mammary glands and nerve-endings are very reactive can increase their sensuality and integrate the energy in the area of the solar plexus and the heart, at the level of the 3rd and 4th chakras.

ACCEPTING OUR OWN EMOTIONS

When we repress an emotion, we are depriving ourselves of untold wealth. Restraining a desire to scream or cry, for example. Keeping our pain to ourselves out of pride. Programmed by our upbringing or by society, we are often unable to express our love or show our pleasure, possibly also for fear of being rejected. Restraint with the goal of letting nothing show will ultimately snuff out the possibility of any true intimacy. To say nothing of the fact that when the sexual liberation years were over, emotions were again associated with weakness like other "feminine" values.

We often play a role, for example we act the way the other person expects of us or the way we imagine that he or she expects. Our intimacy thus remains superficial since our emotions are repressed, our vulnerability is hidden, and our sexual relations become ritualistic. And this problem begets another, a kind of mental blackmail when we surrender a tiny bit of ourselves: "I'll give him/her this if he/she will give me that" is a cowardly reasoning. Even if it leads to a conflict or a quarrel, be brave: nothing ventured, nothing gained. Coming to terms with ourselves is the best way to evolve. Screams and tears are liberating and a couple may grow closer since they often lead to reconciliation. Be Tantric, be generous! A Tantric massage is a form of reconciliation in which we forgive and forget our partner's distorted and bottled-up attitudes. We become as indulgent as when we've had good sex, but the malaise will return if we do not evolve.

When you're on your own, cuddle yourself to learn to better accept emotions, yours as well as those of others, and encourage yourself to express them.

➤ Sitting cross-legged with sloped shoulders, wrap your arms around your shoulders, close your eyes and rock yourself from side to side.

ACCEPTING THE EMOTIONS OF OTHERS

The Canadian Tantric leader Ma Primo stresses the difficulty of accepting another person's emotions, which are often the same as those we cannot accept in ourselves. We can each go on living in our own bubble with our own pretenses or else accept our emotions and express them, open up to what we feel and to our vibrations. If we never vibrate, then we should ask ourselves: "Am I capable of indulging in a bout of melancholy? Under what circumstances?" Repressing negative feelings is not something that stimulates our energy. Better to blow off steam, go jogging, sing or scream (alone) rather than fly into a rage causing a regular hemorrhage of energy which attacks the chi (Chinese word for vital energy) of the liver and by rebound diminishes the vitality of the person near you subjected to your anger.

THE OBSTACLES

In order to take full pleasure in tantric practices such as massage, it is important to rid ourselves of attitudes that are holding us back. This is easier than we might suppose: it will suffice to observe what is actually happening inside of us to modify the alienating forces which we endure.

1. Negative thoughts

Among the long list of toxins that we inject into ourselves, the belief that we have an unsightly body is an especially powerful inhibitor. And yet there is no connection between sexual pleasure and the fact of having a pair of small or sagging breasts, scars, a small penis, a potbelly or cellulitis. We possess all the keys to pleasure, the desire and the intention to take it. Say to yourself: "I am a unique, lovable person and I attract adorable people" or "I like myself the way I am". Saying it over and over again will make it come true. Let the negative thoughts float across your mind like clouds in the sky.

2. The radio in our head

By dint of always being on the qui vive, coping with several things at once and permanently connected to the whole world, our adrenaline becomes a drug. Many of us are addicted to corrosive hyperactivity. Our mind is monopolized by a succession of unrelated thoughts. The coming week's diary runs through our head while we are making love.

Just becoming aware of invasive thoughts is a great step forward. For example, to realize "here I am thinking about work while I'm making love" or "damn it, that's the third time I've gone over those possibilities". Looking for answers to the questions that confront you, making plans for the future, all of that can wait. Concentrating on our breathing short-circuits our thoughts. It is a way of returning to the present when we can't keep them from droning on and on. Our sensations, the feel of the caresses we receive, the warmth of a beloved body close to ours, we are filled with the awareness of this unique moment. Here and now.

3. Stress

At the end of a stressful day, sex often is used to go to sleep. It becomes mechanical. Each partner is locked into their stream of conscious, inside their bubble. In an existence ruled by stress, our feverish mental activity uses up energy, including the energy stored in the sacrum. Stress clouds our perceptions and sometimes prevents us from seeing a love relation as it really is and what it brings us, evaluating our true sexual needs.

Chapter 4

BREATHING

Air is our greatest source of energy, the fuel for our organs and joints. Become aware of the importance of breathing: if we could unfold the air cells in our lungs and spread them out on the ground, they would cover a tennis court. Hunched over our computers, we have gotten into the bad habit of taking in just enough air to stay alive, which lowers our sensitivity to what is around us and to ourselves. Perhaps indeed we are breathing in slow motion and little puffs precisely to protect ourselves from the outside world. According to the New York sexologist Barbara Carrellas (*Urban Tantra*), this is a cultural phenomenon. On the other hand, as soon as we fill our lungs, we are connected with ourselves and with others. The sensation of being alive is as sharp as if we were dancing. People who exhale more easily than they inhale often have difficulty receiving. Breathing properly drives out the fears that haunt us. We learn how to control our breathing by experience, like pearl divers at the bottom of the sea.

BREATHING IS AN INTERNAL MASSAGE

CONSCIOUS BREATHING

Spend a few minutes every day, getting some fresh air into your lungs and emptying your mind with these breathing techniques. As soon as your mental radio shuts down, you begin to yawn: this is the sign that you are relaxing. In Yoga as in a Tantric massage, the body acts on the mind. By dint of being permanently connected with the whole world, our mind is constantly monopolized by various thoughts. Emptying it out means letting all those thoughts run through it without focusing on any single one until they disappear completely. That is when peace sets in.

This breathing purge prevents negative thoughts from polluting you; negative thoughts such as resentment, jealousy or anger (it blocks the liver), anxiety (it perturbs the spleen), sadness, defeatist attitudes and sorrow (all harmful for the lungs), erode your overall energy potential and your sexual power. They no longer affect you when you concentrate on your breathing. The mental has a great deal of power over the physical, as is shown by psychosomatic disorders. It is up to us to reverse this process: our body will guide our mind by our conscious breathing.

BREATHING THROUGH THE NOSE

When you breathe through the nose your parasympathetic system lowers your blood pressure and slows your heartbeat. If you attend to your breathing and nothing else, you will soon feel soothed. This is the breathing associated with Yoga and meditation.

➤ Sitting cross-legged, stretch the skin on your buttocks to the rear in order to open the chakras and line them up with the sacrum. Your shoulders droop, your armpits are open, the top of your head is connected with the ceiling by an invisible thread, your tongue lies flaccidly on your palate. All we do is concentrate on the breath that lies at the center of the heart. Little by little, your breathing becomes more refined, more protracted and extremely subtle, and the chakras awaken.

The different kinds of active breathing can be practiced several times a day when you have a few minutes to yourself. These breathing techniques trigger an internal alchemy which aimed at purifying and magnetizing the spinal column and stimulating the nervous system. By opening up the channels between the chakras, they put us back in touch with our true essence, the fundamental unity in which all Asians believe, irrespective of the existential drama of each individual. They also make it possible to diminish or even eliminate the stress which prevents us from living the present moment to the hilt.

1. TOTAL BREATHING

— Sitting cross-legged, the skin on your buttocks drawn back and your anus exposed as in all these positions, inhale with your stomach for five seconds: bring the air up into your solar plexus, then to your clavicles as though you were inflating a balloon.

— Pull your shoulders up so as to fill your lungs to the brim.

— Hold your breath for five seconds. Inhale again. This liberates tension and favors exhalation.

— Breathe through the nose slowly.

Begin again 10 times over. This total breathing massages all your organs and arouses your sleeping vital energy, enabling it to irrigate your organs and your chakras.

2. BUMBLEBEE BREATHING

— Sit on the floor. Ideally, for a good cleansing, you should sit cross-legged with bowed torso and your forehead lying on your fists placed one on top of the other on the floor, thumbs in palms and neck muscles relaxed.

— If you are not flexible enough for this, sit on your heels with your legs folded under you, and bend forward to your fists on the floor as above.

Breathe through the nose while keeping this position, thus releasing all your mental agitation into the floor. Make this position even more powerful by buzzing like a bumblebee for several minutes.

3. Orbital breathing (seated or standing)

This internal solo massage can be practiced anywhere, for example instead of a coffee break, to improve your dynamic.

- Place your hands on your belly, index fingers joined above the pubis, thumbs on the navel. Your fingers should form a triangle. The tip of your tongue should be touching your palate just behind the incisors as in most Tantra or Taichi sequences. This way, the path followed by the chi or vital breath describes a closed loop which travels up the spinal column and down the front of you via the tongue and the throat to the navel.
- Breathe through the nose. The energy, the breath, the chi starts from the dantian just beneath the navel, travels down to the perineum during exhalation, then travels up the spinal column, the back of the head and over the top of the skull, down to the palate, and via the throat to the perineum, then back up the spinal column.

At first you may feel nothing. But if you persevere, you will start to localize the energy circulating in this orbit by concentrating on the path it follows and imagining that your breath is moving along this circuit. This simple but powerful exercise makes it possible to activate the sexual energy that lies sleeping at the base of your spinal column, the kundalinî already discussed.

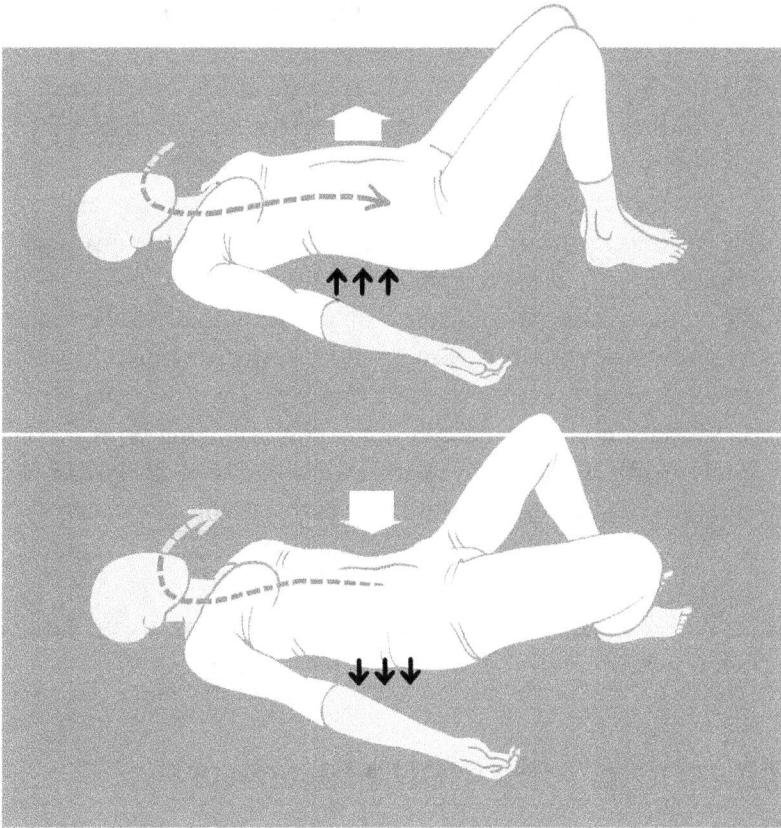

2. Undulatory orbital breathing

4. Undulatory orbital breathing (in a prone position)

— Lie down with your legs tucked up and spread the width of your pelvis, feet flat on the floor, arms stretched out on either side of your body, palms turned up. Your tongue is pressed to your palate just behind the incisors.

— Inhale deeply through the nose with your anus and your navel protruding and your pelvis pressed to the floor. You feel the air inflating your stomach.

At the end of the breathing, bring your pelvis slightly higher by contracting your PC muscle (anus and perineum) and your thighs. Your body ripples like a wave, slowly.

— In the same position, imagine that your whole body opens up to receive the breath you inhale. Energy is being diffused through your organs and your muscles as you breathe. Try to identify with your breathing by concentrating on it. Feel your breath, the chi, circulating through your body like a slow electric current, and guide it towards your abdomen as you breathe out, no longer pressing your knees together and relaxing your anus.

The ebb and flow of your breath revitalize your organs and massages them, energizing all the chakras on the way.

BREATHING THROUGH THE MOUTH

1. Athletic breathing

Breathing in through the mouth during an outdoor athletic activity such as jogging or cycling allows us to store up more oxygen and refuel our body.

2. Yang breathing

When you feel tense, breathe through the mouth. This will drive out the fire, the surplus of yang piled up in your thorax and head because of your stress... because of holding your breath over your computer. Breathing out through the mouth makes it easier to get rid of the tension and to let go. The Japanese shout during their martial arts sessions, in karate for example, tightening their muscles to speed up their metabolism. In the Tantra, we generally breathe out through the mouth.

3. Misty exhaling

Breathe in through the nose and breathe out very slowly and silently with your mouth scarcely open, as though you were trying to fog up a mirror. This type of breathing gently relaxes the diaphragm.

CHAPTER 5

BALANCING
OUR CHAKRAS

"Chakra means wheel. It's like a potter's wheel. If you step on the pedal, the wheel turns, if you don't step on it, the wheel remains still. In other words, we have no chakras if we don't make them turn," (Daniel Odier, *Tantra*). The seven chakras listed here are energy points located up and down the body, between the sacrum and the top of the cranium. Our knowledge of the chakras, those loci of energy transformation and exchange —of which there are many more minor ones— derives from Hindu philosophy. We might also call them by their Chinese names, since they correspond to the pressure points of Chinese medicine. The chi (vital energy), called prana by the Indians, nourishes our vital centers and may be stimulated by techniques of acupuncture applied to certain reflex points. Each of these has its own vibratory qualities: they are vibrational nodules. The fourth chakra, the sexual chakra, opens up when the lower part of the body is massaged (abdomen, sacrum, pubis, genitals). Our mind has the power to act upon our chakras. Bringing our chakras into line and balancing them is accomplished by visualizing the colors of the rainbow and their vibrations. The techniques of visualization suggested below after the description of the specificities of each chakra will help you to get in closer touch with yourself. Working on one's chakras is a plus if we want to achieve the self-knowledge which is an indispensable part of Tantrism.

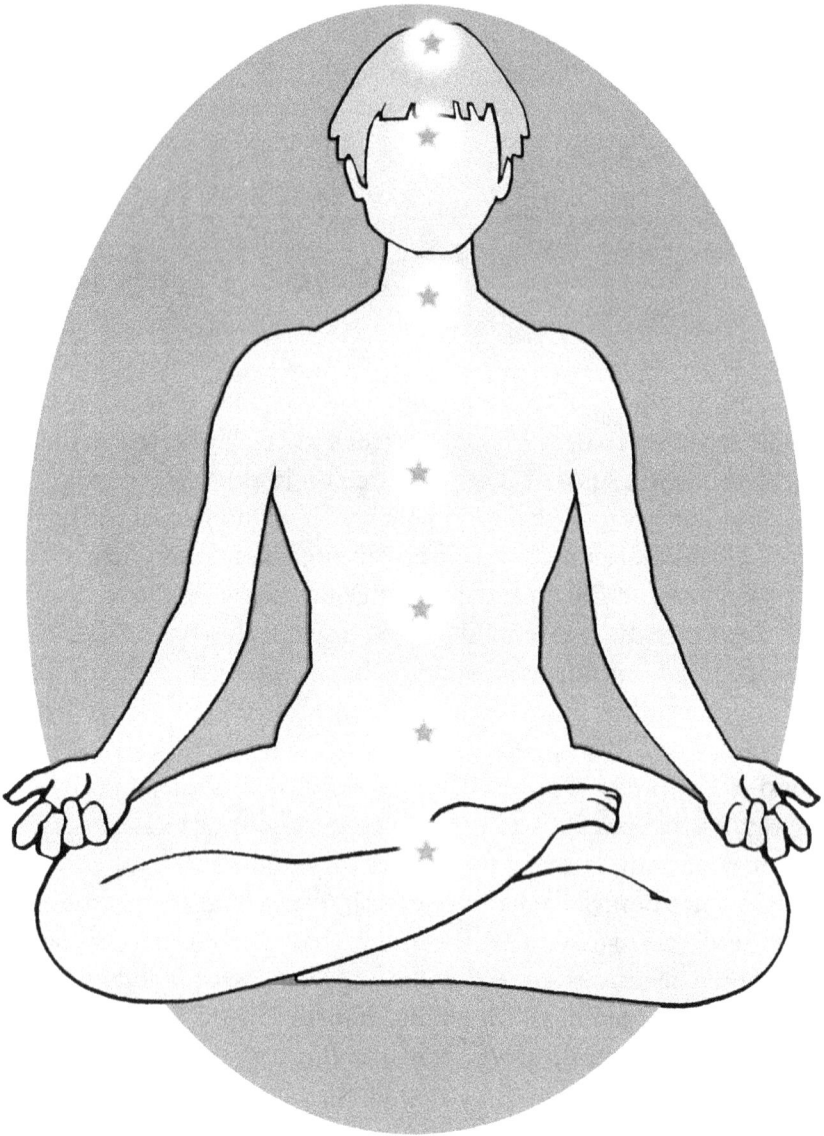

3. The 7 main chakras.

TANTRIC AND KASHMIRI MASSAGES

THE FIRST CHAKRA

THE ROOT CENTER

Corresponding motives

Color: deep red.
Body area: feet, sacrum, rectum, immune system.
Metaphysical: rootedness, survival, self-confidence, security, solidity and stability, the unconscious.

Located between the anus and the genitals, it contains our latent male/female energy: it is the seat of the kundalinî at the base of the spine. It is linked with death and the fear of loss, which it also allows us to overcome. The Chinese give the name Jen Mo to the most external and most sensitive part of the prostate gland. In alchemy, we speak of a sacred fire originating in the sacrum: it is the root center of sexual energy at the base of the spine, our coccyx corresponds to the tail which enables animals to keep their balance and links us to the earth. The inability to reach orgasm is often the result of a lack of rootedness: people who cannot reach orgasm are cut off by conditioning from their environment, especially if they were an undesired or ill-treated child. This chakra is also associated with the family, the group, the tribe, survival, whatever we own, money symbolizing security and the reproduction of the species.

Meditation

To meditate on this chakra, concentrate on your sacrum while visualizing the color red. Make the red field rotate, trying to feel the heat it gives off. Think about the emotional releases in your past life or in the present and try to combine them with the revolving red. After a while your feelings will be clarified and better balanced.

To balance this chakra you can also:

- Imagine that your spine has roots going down to the center of the earth and keep this feeling of rootedness while sitting somewhere.
- Go walking in a natural environment
- Stamp your foot
- Run
- Dance, the belly dance or some African dance, for example
- Massage your perineum (see **Chapter 20**)
- Take up Qigong or Taichi.

THE SECOND CHAKRA

THE CENTER OF PLEASURE, OF OUR PHYSICAL ORIGIN, OF THE SYMPHONY OF LIFE

Corresponding motives

Color: orange.
Body area: pelvis, ovaries, uterus, prostate and testicles, kidneys and adrenal glands bones, sense of hearing.
Metaphysical: the awakening of sexuality, pleasure, physical energy, the instinctive insights of our senses.

Located three finger-widths below the naval, this point, the dantian in Chinese, also called "the fountain of life", is where our vital energy (chi) is stored and whence our feelings, pleasant or unpleasant, radiate.

It is the center of reproduction. It governs our physical and emotional drives, both sexual and creative. The emotions linked to our relations with others such as fear or jealousy are disseminated to the other chakras and to our organs from this second brain, that of our "gut feelings". Today we know that the millions of neurons located in our intestines constitute our stress-sensitive second brain. It is symbolized by an archer taking aim at a target.

The second chakra is also linked with the powers we are subjected to and with whatever these powers —patriarchal, matriarchal or societal— inflict upon us: there is always some taboo which we take pleasure in breaking. The fear of being seen masturbating is a mark of stigmatization by authorities that repress youth: parents, school, society, religion, laws. The difficulties of self-fulfillment or getting an erection are linked with that. Sex and money are also associated with this chakra: increased earnings often heighten our sexual appetite.

Meditation

To meditate on the second chakra, you will make the color orange appear two centimeters below your naval and set it in rotation. If you encounter difficulties visualizing that color, think of an orange, for instance. Your meditation will dilute your negative attitudes in that orange light, including the fear of not being creative or unproductive.

To balance this chakra you may also:

- Concentrate on this point while breathing deeply
- Talk about sex with friends
- Arrange to have a deep tissue massage or an acupuncture session
- Eroticize your breathing by yourself (see orbital breathing, end of **Chapter 4**)
- Maintain a powerfully emotive contact with nature
- Play with huge bursts of laughter
- Roar like a wild beast

THE THIRD CHAKRA

THE CENTER OF POWER, THE EGO AND SENSIBILITY

Corresponding motives

Color: yellow.

Body area: stomach, pancreas, the liver and its influence on the eyes, the large intestine.

Metaphysical: identity, confidence, peace, self-satisfaction and self-esteem, courage, kindness, thirst for power and possession, intense activity.

Located in the solar plexus, this is the center of our personal power, our ability to find our place in the world, a territory close to what we truly are. If we position ourselves as a dominant person or as a victim, if we divide the world between winners and losers, then this chakra is not balanced. We are likely to have behavioral problems and offload them onto others, or take love as a pretext to avoid seeing a relationship as it really is. Our lack of self-confidence is likely to stifle the frightening emotions that come with having sex. This may be the result of adults having failed to lend you a sympathetic ear during a difficult childhood.

Meditation

To meditate on this chakra, let your solar plexus bathe in sunshine yellow until all tension has gone out of it. The vibrations of emotional disorder will dissolve into the color yellow, including your fear of losing some thing, some person or some part of yourself intimately linked with your ego. By meditating on the third chakra, you will ultimately like yourself better.

To balance this chakra you may also:

- Talk to yourself out loud in front of a mirror, adumbrating the qualities which you recognize in yourself
- Laugh very loudly
- Take up a martial art
- Have someone massage your feet
- Punch a pillow

THE FOURTH CHAKRA

THE CENTER OF LOVE, OF ONESELF AND OF OTHERS

Corresponding motives

Color: green.
Body area: thymus, heart, chest, breasts, lungs, arms and hands, tongue (sense of taste).
Metaphysical: love and compassion, emotions, intuition, opening, intimacy, joy, honor, enthusiasm, radiance, sincerity, but also impatience, cruelty and violence.

This is the chakra of the qualities of heart: love, generosity, ability to forgive. Love depends on our capacity to be moved, to experience wonder at the beauties of nature and the sex act. It is a force stronger than ego. In a balanced sexual relationship, we give at least as much as we receive. Opening our heart means communication and sharing. A heart condition is often due to a conflict between our feelings and our mind. A lung condition related to resentment and sadness that can be fought against by sending out positive energy, in particular, for a woman, by massaging her breasts. This point is the bridge between the physical (the three lower chakras) and the mental (the three upper ones).

Meditation

To meditate on this chakra, visualize the color green at the level of your heart and make it revolve, thus stimulating the management of your feelings and your endocrine system. Irradiation through the love drive – via the heart – can heal the whole body. The color green is soothing and can neutralize a fit of rage.

To balance this chakra you may also:

- Concentrate on your breathing
- Massage your breasts – in a woman, this can arouse compassion and love
- Emit a long chant "Aaah!" holding open palms towards the sky
- Examine what's wrong with you and have a good cry

Fifth chakra

THE CENTER OF VERBAL EXPRESSION

Corresponding motives

Color: blue.
Body areas: throat, neck, thyroid, mouth, teeth, ears.
Metaphysical: communication, voice expression, creativity, choice.

This is the center of creation and communication. The resonance of pleasure should make the throat vibrate in a chant of pleasure rising from the genitals. Expressing the unspoken, communicating in the sex act correspond to the thyroid gland which regulates the sexual function via your hormones. This is also the center of willpower, of addiction to drugs, spirits or sex. Frequent sore throats or toothache can be linked with problems of willpower, communication or addiction.

Meditation

To meditate on this chakra, try to understand the reasons for a feeling of resentment which keeps you chained to some unconscious fear. By giving it up, you make room for positive feelings: love provides the most delightful channel of communication. Meditating on the blue chakra in the throat will eliminate a possible blockage. If you need to talk to someone about a problem, mix the colors blue and green to put your heart into it. This color may be used whenever you have something hard to say to someone.

To balance this chakra you may also:

- Sing, join a choir
- Bill and coo or sing with a partner
- Join a theater group
- Opt for some creative activity
- Meditate

THE SIXTH CHAKRA

THE CENTER OF INNER VISION, OF THE IMAGINATION AND THE AWAKENING OF CONSCIOUSNESS

Corresponding motives

Color: silver blue (the color of the moon).
Body areas: the eyes and the pineal gland which governs your other glands and your metabolism.
Metaphysical: memory, intuition, imagination, good sense, forgiveness, capacity to see yourself as you really are, spiritual experiences, telepathy.

Located in the center of the forehead between the eyes, this point is also known as the third eye. It allows you to see yourself with precision. Its power increases in proportion with the healing of those wounds standing in the way of our lucidity. People who develop their insights nourish their sixth chakra, opening it to imagination, dreams and colored visions. They increase their reactive powers in every area, including sex.

Meditation

To meditate on this chakra, concentrate on the third eye in the middle of your forehead. This meditation is appropriate when you wish to manifest some aspect of yourself, project a facet of your being.

To balance this chakra, you may also:

- Sleep out of doors
- Increase your exposure to daylight or a sunlamp
- Go in for introspection, act as a witness of yourself, your innermost thoughts, your reactions and your emotions
- Have your feet massaged
- Train your memory by contemplating some object and then recalling it with your eyes closed.

The seventh chakra

THE SPIRITUAL CENTER

Corresponding motives

Color: white.
Body areas: brain, hypothalamus, central nervous system.
Metaphysical: attention, ecstasy, the higher form of Love, spirituality, consciousness, mindfulness (the spiritual seventh heaven).

This is where kings wear their crowns and is in fact called "the crown" in the Tantra, our antenna towards the spiritual, the halo of saints. It is our awakening, our connection with the collective unconscious, but also the center of mindfulness as well as the awareness of all things. When this chakra is blocked, everything goes dark inside and around us. One often speaks of the sacred with respect to the crown, but this does not mean that this chakra has anything to do with religion: to have a high esteem for humanity and for nature is to regard them as sacred. When we have a complete orgasm, this chakra opens wide. When energy rises in the moment of relaxation after an orgasm, the two poles, the yin and the yang are fused into one.

Meditation

To meditate on this chakra, the color violet will oscillate faster than others, try to visualize it as a long tongue of flame rising within you. You may also visualize a white light exploding over your head, or else place yourself inside a white bubble. These visualizations connected with the chakra crown facilitate your access to the spiritual plane of everything, including love.

To balance this chakra, you may also:

- Have orgasms
- Pretend to die
- Massage or brush your scalp
- Undergo an Ayurvedic Sirodhara (pouring warm oil on your forehead while you lie on your back)
- Meditate

Chapter 6

NUDITY AND THE ART OF TOUCH

NUDITY

THE NUDITY OF INNOCENCE

That is the state of mind in which to approach holistic massage between a couple or in a one-off exchange. You are strongly advised to massage the entire body or let yourself be massaged all over, even if the genitals are left untouched in the course of a first massage: this can be decided in a preliminary conversation. If the receiver is a man and he has an erection during the massage, the man or woman massaging him must not be offended. Choosing a giver of your own sex is sometimes important if you are timid or prudish. Some prefer being massaged by a person of the opposite sex in order to receive a different kind of charge, feminine (yin) from a woman or masculine (yang) from a man.

NAKEDNESS TO RECONCILE YOURSELF WITH YOUR OWN IMAGE

In the last analysis, a Tantric masseur/euse is the benevolent mirror that you decide to allow yourself since you are exhibiting yourself to yourself. Getting to love our body nourishes a Tantric massage, self-love is a precondition for any true love of others. It is in fact one of the objectives of the massage: afterwards, being naked will no longer seem a problem to you.

It is important to free yourself from the shame of nakedness which our societies impose on us, all the more so as while the Tantra is now as popular as the New Age movement in the eighties, Mary Whitehouse is back again, proof that the entire world is still taking its cue from the Anglo-Saxons and letting them set the pace. In the Western world, prudery always returns in cycles. Renaissance painters portrayed women in low-cut gowns. Not so long ago, the topless fashion on beaches was a sign of sexual liberation, but times have changed: nudity today is considered a provocation as it was in the fifties. In India, it has been outlawed ever since medieval Islam (and the arrival of the Protestant colonizers), which means that today massages are reserved for foreigners.

NAKEDNESS OF THE RECEIVER

If it is a one-time massage, receivers are actually often less embarrassed by their nakedness in front of a stranger whom they might never see again than in a lasting relationship. However, some people feel embarrassed exposing nakedness to another person whoever it might be. Moreover, our relationship to our body grows more uncomfortable as we grow older... or gain weight. Consequently, the increased awareness of our body and its imperfections and the shame that follows seems to be increasing in a period of exhibitionism and narcissism.

NUDITY IS ECOLOGICAL

From a purely practical point of view, nakedness has the advantage of allowing an oil-massage without having pounds of various clothing to wash afterwards. After an Ayurvedic massage, the sarong that the giver uses to cover the parts of the body which are not being dealt with is stiff and heavy with oil.

The g-string

Prior to a Tantric massage, a health spa will offer customers a disposable g-string thus sparing them the inconvenience of tight knickers or underpants out of consideration for the modesty of both participants in such a "commercial" establishment. Independent professionals sometimes provide the same type of disposable underwear. However, most of them recommend complete nudity in order to benefit from a complete range of sensations. When we are naked, we can get to the bottom of ourselves, enjoy wholeheartedly the slippery, sensual effect of the oil and the giver's palms on our skin.

Nakedness of the giver

In a health spa, the masseurs are fully dressed as in any massage parlor and work around the receiver lying down on a massage table. An independent masseur or masseuse is often wearing only panties, a pair of shorts or a swimsuit in order to avoid brushing against the customer with their genitals, whether the massage is being carried out on a table or on the floor. Some female Tantric practitioners wear a swimsuit top to make sure their breasts do not bob about on the receiver's body when she bends over them.

THE ART OF TOUCHING

A massage acts on some of the 640,000 tactile receptors connected to the spinal cord and the brain by half a million nerves. Touch is the core of massage. It stimulates the hypothalamus, at the back of the brain, and causes a general parasympathetic unwinding of our muscles, an incomparable mode of relaxation.

Massage is perhaps the most potent exchange that exists between two human beings. It allows for a contact with another person who is a perfect stranger. The skin is our relational organ, another way of getting to know someone via the sense of touch, a massage strengthens our immunologic defenses and hormonal production, cures insomnia, resolves stress and aggressiveness, lowers blood pressure and slows the heartbeat. It acts more efficiently on the emotional brain than a conversation, all the more so in a Tantric massage as the massaging hands are charged with love.

When giving a massage, concentrate on your hands:

They are generally lying flat with fingers together, or cupped during a pause. Fill them with love. If you have feelings of self-doubt, choose a method you can remember, from a massage you have received, adapting it to the sensibility of your partner. For some a touch that is too light (a yin touch) will feel as if you were tickling them. But an overly firm touch (a yang touch) will prevent other people from letting go. Don't be afraid to ask your partner if what you are doing suits them. Adapt your movements accordingly.

No hurry

Slowness is the distinctive mark of a Tantric massage, it is tantamount to a yoga of the touch which addresses the body as a whole. Completely different from the techniques of Ayurvedic massage which jostle the whole body, passing vigorously time and again over the limbs and joints, studiously avoiding the genitals.

THE YIN TOUCH

This is used at the beginning and/or the end of a Tantric massage. It consists in brushing your fingers lightly over the subject's skin or slowly sliding your palm without exerting the slightest pressure and yet with no suggestion of tickling. The palm, the fingers (or fingertips) slide slowly and delicately. Using a silky fabric or feathers may heighten the effect of the yin touch.

THE YANG TOUCH

The most commonly used technique for a Tantric massage. Its firmness allows you to penetrate deeply, to resolve tensions, enter the fasciae and reach the neuro-vegetative system. Kneading, sliding, pinching, describing large and small circles with a firm yang type pressure of the fingers, the thumb alone, the whole palm with joined fingers and often, with the heel of the hand. The yang touch is used in the integration phase of the massage of a given part of the body in order to energize it.

THE MEDITATIVE TOUCH

This is used like a freeze frame in a movie, your hands are resting on two different points of the body you are massaging, hands lying flat on two distant chakras: an ankle or a wrist, the subject's heart and head, etc. There must be no intentionality in your hands, only love.

THE DEEP TOUCH

When you lay your hands for the first time on the body of your receiver or during a pause in the massage, give depth to your touch. It can be penetrating and yet with no intention. It is a matter of your presence to the Other and to yourself, a presence to the moment and to the touch.

No matter which touch you choose, your awareness brings your energy and benevolent attention into your hands.

SOLO EXERCISE TO IMPROVE YOUR TOUCH

BECOME AWARE OF YOUR OWN BODY

This technique is borrowed from Eutonia, a method invented by a Germano-Danish woman, Gerda Alexander, aimed at ridding the body of harmful habits and persistent tensions. It consists of awakening our perceptions of our body to relax it and feel more positive about ourself. A better awareness of our own body can help us lend a sympathetic ear to another person... and to oneself.

By rolling a tennis ball over your body lightly, you will feel how the skin defines its limits. By exerting a little pressure on the ball, you will feel your muscles. You can also lie on the ground or on a carpet and roll it under your body, lying first on one side, then the other. This work on your sense of touch can de profitable for anyone interested in this type of massage.

SELF-MASSAGE

Here the objective is to discover yourself, to feel the sensibility of your own skin, to calibrate and refine the way you touch it. It is best to practice this massage of an evening, in the quiet of your own home.

With soft music and good vapors from a diffuser of essential oils, lie face down in the Yoga svastika posture which will open your heart (see **Chapter 3**). Hold this position for a nourishing 10 minutes. Now take a foetal position in order to make the gradual transition to lying prone on your back.

First recharge your energy batteries using the method devised by the sino-thai doctor Mantak Chia (see karsai self-massage, **Chapter 18**). Then sit cross-legged. Massage your face with the fingertips of both hands, from the wings of your nose to your hairline. Massage once around each eye from the bottom of the dark ring towards the nose and outwards. Pinch your eyebrows between thumb and forefinger. Press insistently with the whole length of one forefinger on the space between you upper lip and your nose, then under the lower lip. Rub your fingertips on your scalp at the top of your skull, then behind your ears, from top to bottom, symmetrically. Finish off by massaging your ears with the tips of your forefingers, tugging at the lobes in a final gesture.

Next you massage your hands without any oil, by pressing the thumb of the other hand into the center of the palm, varying the degree of pressure to gauge the difference. Switch from a yin touch to a yang touch. Massage each finger, kneading it slowly, with special attention to the joints. Move slowly up the outside of the forearm past the elbow to he shoulder, wrap your fingers around the arm and proceed back down to the fingertips. Take advantage of this to try different techniques on yourself, pressing with the heel of the hand in a light sliding motion with varying pressures. Practice the slow tempo characteristic of the Tantra. Finish off with the same enveloping movement but only just touching your arm.

THE DIFFERENT MASSAGE TECHNIQUES

SLIDING

This is the most common technique in a Tantric massage. It is used on the back, the sides, the arms and legs, the torso and the buttocks. Oil your hands copiously in order to achieve the toboggan effect and cover a large surface of the prone body in a single slow slide. Count some 8 to 10 seconds from the neck to the buttocks, for example. Maintain an even, light pressure with the whole hand, fingers together. When you carry out a long sliding movement, let the weight of your body propel your hands forward, even if it means rising up on your knees. Repeat each sliding movement two or three times. When you use a lighter (yin) touch, the sliding may be curved or wavy.

The different pressures:

- Heavy
- Light
- Varied, with the whole hand, fingers joined
- With the heel of the hand
- With the fingers
- Stretching the receiver's body
- Lifting their hips or pelvis

These pressures are applied with supple fingers: no pinching. Nor should you seize handfuls of flesh except for the kneading-rolling technique, which is seldom used in this kind of massage.

BROAD CIRCLES

Your hands work outwards in opposite directions. They follow identical divergent paths and come together again at the starting point. This generally begins with a downward movement and then upwards in a straight line. It is used on the receiver's back when they are lying face down. Your hands move down the back and up the sides. You may also describe circles on the receiver's buttocks, starting at the bottom of their back.

KNEADING

This touch is meant to deal with the deep tissues and muscles: you grip them with your whole hand and knead them as you would bread dough. You squeeze the fleshy parts (back, buttocks, sides) between your thumb and fingers, then release. Your hands may also take turns kneading, squeezing the flesh, alternately and symmetrically. Kneading is often used to deal with knotted muscles in the shoulders and upper back in order to unwind the receiver's stress at the beginning of a massage. It is rarely used in a meditative or emotional style massage.

THE LIGHT TOUCH

Using your fingertips, place your partner in a state of receptivity without rushing them. This "yin touch" may be used at the beginning or the end of a massage to awaken the receiver's sensuality or in alternation with a firmer touch. A very slow, light touch creates an erotic sensation in the neck, the hips, the pubis and genitals. They bring our sensuality to the surface of the skin.

At the beginning of a massage, brush your fingers up and down the receiver's back. Then focus on the nape of the neck and shoulders, describing circles with your fingertips.

If this light touch is used to finish the massage, the receiver is lying on their back. Brush your fingers down their body from neck to ankles, then the torso, drawing tighter and tighter clockwise circles on their belly, ending with tiny circles around their naval.

Let your hand rest motionless before you break contact. Alternatively: you may also run your fingers down their legs, from crotch to instep, at least two or three times at the end of the massage, and leave their body at the big toe, the way a bird takes flight.

KNEADING-ROLLING

Pinch with moderate pressure the receiver's skin between thumb and forefinger (or two or three fingers) moving them down their back or sides. Actually this technique is mainly used on a woman's labia during a Tantric sexual massage or on a receiver well versed in the Tantra. Other than these two examples, this technique is seldom used in a Tantric massage.

PINCER

Your hand is used like a pair of tongs to seize an extremity, for example all of the toes. Or else to seize one finger and slide to the tip before letting go. The pincer is composed of the three longest fingers and the thumb, and is used to squeeze and then release its grip while pulling gently as if to limber up a member.

CHAPTER 7

EXERCISES FOR TWO

For beginners in Tantric massage, certain exercises for two will enable them to familiarize themselves with direct physical contact. In a Tantric learning session we are taught how to approach a partner's body, their energy and spirituality and also how to touch them. These exercises are quite simple. But if we take them seriously they can be very rewarding. Each of them lasts about 10 minutes and involves no talking.

THE WHO-AM-I?

Sitting cross-legged face to face or standing a half-meter apart, we look into each other's eyes asking our partner "Who am I?" but without actually speaking the words. It will make us feel slightly uncomfortable when two partners who do not know each other stare into each other's eyes before starting a massage. When the "Who-Am-I" is practiced frequently, the partners may succeed in actually becoming one during rare moments.

The "Who-Am-I" on one's own
Practiced on one's own as was advocated by Maharsi, one of the great Hindu masters of the 20th century,

the "who-am-I" causes fear, uncertainty and ultimately "a state of silent clear-headedness as if nothing can exist outside of this "I am". Through it the world will appear" (Jean Klein, *I am*). Our habit of personifying our image, the ego, will tend to disappear at the end of this exercise. Our mind faces a void. We arrive at "I am" by preventing our consciousness from clinging to any qualification whatsoever.

FEEL YOUR ENERGIES ABOVE YOUR PARTNER'S BODY

Your partner lies on their back.

- Place your hands 5 centimeters above their body.
  Move them slowly, from the pubis to the top of the head.
- Try to feel the energy differences, some areas are warm and vibrant, others are cold and inert.
- Next exchange roles and then tell each other what you have felt, but without exaggeration, you are not play-acting.

If you didn't feel much, don't hesitate to say so. It doesn't matter whether you make any progress or not. The important thing is to be present, firmly in the here and now, taking interest in your body energy and entering into an authentic sharing experience.

MICROMASSAGE

This exercise enables beginners to practice on a partner before trying their hand at an overall massage. It is practiced on bare skin. You familiarize yourself with the use of the oil and how much of it to use at a time. Massaging your partner's forearm or leg is a good way to acquire a feeling for the fluidity of your gestures and calibrate your touch.

- Begin with a single hand, pressing and sliding very slowly.
- Next, massage symmetrically, with one hand on each side of the limb. Avoid a caressing effect as that is not what one expects of a massage, and avoid rubbing, which can be unpleasantly mechanical.
- Learn to feel the difference between a light (yin) touch, which can tickle the receiver or get on their nerves if it is not done right, and the firmness of a sliding pressure (yang touch).
- Start taking 10 to 15 second pauses on a body extremity, one hand resting on the other on your partner's ankle for example. The pressure you apply must be moderately firm. After each pause, the resumption must be slow.
- Avoid putting any intentionality into your touch or dwelling too long on any given area.
- Be attentive to what is happening in the receiver's body.

After a few minutes, exchange roles. Then discuss with complete sincerity what each of you has felt.

A good massage will deepen the sensibility of both partners.

CRADLING THE HEAD

This is a way to experience letting go. One of the partners lies on their back. The other sits on the floor behind their head, supporting its weight in both hands. Being thus gently cradled, the person on their back is no longer in control: their partner has gently taken over and they can offload all their worries. This letting-go will gradually spread to the whole body. The person doing the cradling will end the exercise by placing three fingers on the eyebrows or temples of the person on their back.

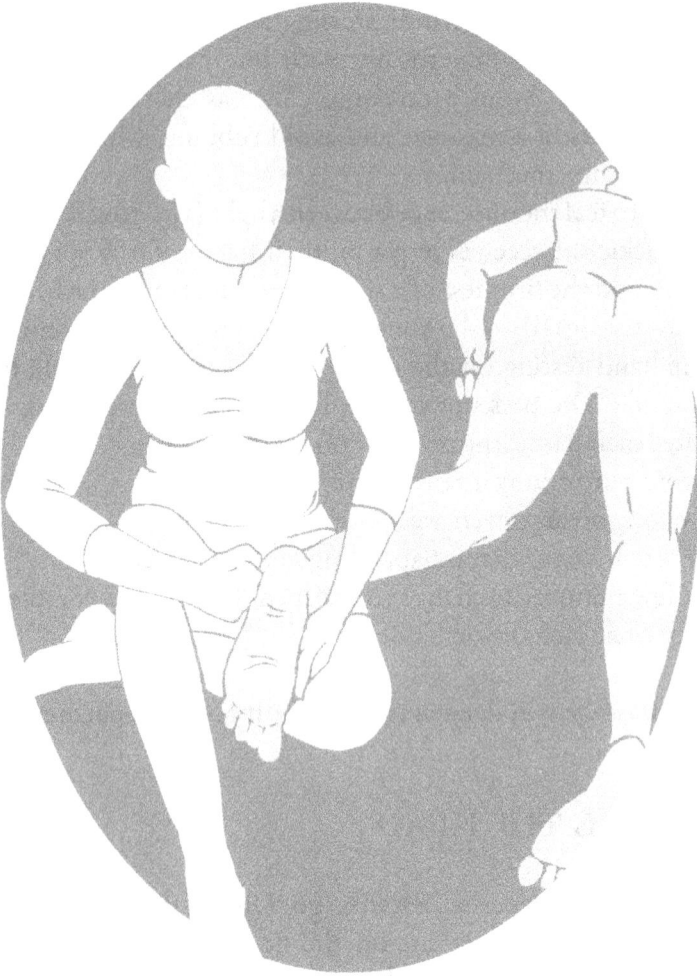

Figure 4. Foot massage.

TANTRIC AND KASHMIRI MASSAGES

BLINDFOLDED

Blindfold first your partner, lying on the floor, and then yourself. Your sensations will be greatly amplified and the quality of your touch improved. This is way of experimenting with your touch as a giver, to have a better grasp of what you are doing because you will be totally concentrated. You will feel with greater accuracy your partner's epidermal reactions. The stimuli provided by your hands should be gradual: begin with the lightest touch, then move up the scale: yin, yang, meditative, deep. Take advantage of this to try out the differing degrees of pressure and the different moves described in **Chapter 6**.

MASSAGES OF SPECIFIC AREAS
Massaging the feet

The receiver is lying on their stomach, the giver sitting cross-legged.

- Take hold of the foot with both hands, bending the knee just a little.
- Massage with one hand the under-side of the outer edge of the foot, towards the center of the sole: the energy reflex point corresponding to our sexuality is located on the sole just behind the pads.
- Dig your thumb three or four times into the hollow there.
- Then massage the sole of the foot, working towards the center, this time concentrating on the inner edge of the arch.
- Squeeze one after another the joints of the toes then pull each toe delicately towards you, the little toe last.
- Finish by massaging upwards, the ankle and the leg.

The resulting relaxation will make your partner very receptive.

A RELAXING KOREAN FACIAL MASSAGE

Kneel behind the head of the person lying on their back with their face between your legs.

- Begin by pressing both sides of their chin in order to loosen their jaw. Thus your partner will be rid of our tendency to snatch, bite, consume.
- Press the tips of your hooked fingers under the cheek-bones to stretch the skin on the cheeks towards the ears, then brush your hands over the face from the chin to the temples.
- Do this again exerting more pressure. This way you will facilitate the irrigation of the ears and the optic nerve.
- Slide your finger pads from the wings of the nose to the ears, smoothing the face. The receiver becomes aware of their mask and finds inner peace.
- Place both thumbs between the eyebrows and slide them to the ears to alleviate the worry-related tensions.
- Press two fingers on the base of the nose, then on the inner corners of the eyes, symmetrically, which creates the effect of clearing the brain, then at the base of the wings of the nose to clear the sinuses.
- Lay your cupped hands over the eyes to diffuse their energy. Finish by describing circles with two or three fingers, from chin to forehead, then decreasing the pressure to the point where you are only brushing over the skin.

CHAPTER 8

GETTING READY FOR A MASSAGE

This oil massage is carried out on the floor, as a deep resonance at heart-level is difficult to obtain when lying on a table: the two bodies' proximity is essential for an intuitive touch. In a setting that is easy on the eyes, you squat on your heels in order to move on your knees around the receiver's body later on. If squatting on your heels hurts your knees or your thighs, you may need a low prayer stool to be comfortable.

CREATE A SUITABLE AMBIANCE

Under a subdued lighting, the surroundings should be pleasant to look at since this type of massage is meant to please all the senses. Choose an ethereal music for its relaxing effect, though the idea is not to go to sleep! Calculate the music you will be playing according to the length of the massage. Use a fragrance dispenser to fill the air with a pleasant scent as burning incense is not so good for your health. You may need a small heater if the room is cold: a body covered with oil feels chilly as if it had just come out of water. The ideal room temperature is around 26-28 ° C.

HOUSEHOLD TEXTILES

Pad the floor with a duvet covered with beach towels which you'd better protect with a big plastic sheet if you are going to use lots of oil to facilitate long sliding moves. This leatherette or oilcloth can be laid over the towels or directly over the duvet.

Have a bath sheet ready to cover them at the end of the massage to let it sink in. Toweling and slippers or a pair of socks will prevent soiling the floor with oil. In winter, a bathrobe is preferable. It is essential to provide a shower facility so that your partner can wash off the oil before getting dressed.

ALL ABOUT MASSAGE OIL

Our sense of smell is connected with the first chakra and is rooted in our primal being. As a source of pleasant aquatic sensations, oil brings us back to childhood, when our mother rubbed and stroked our skin to nourish it. A pleasant scent has the power to awaken our sensuality and release all types of emotions. It take us on a flower-scented journey, elevating the massage to a spiritual plane.

Make your own mixture using natural oils. For example 10% deodorized coconut oil with 90% sunflower or rapeseed oil. Add a few drops of some essential oil: ylang-ylang is said to be aphrodisiac, sandalwood oil has a calming effect on the mind, lemonwood or rosemary oil a purifying effect. Rule out the greasy sesame oil used in Ayurvedic massage as well as carcinogenic petroleum based mineral oils like the notorious "baby oil": Our skin is highly permeable to all the substances we apply to it, no matter if they are salutary or harmful.

How much oil should we use?

There are several schools. Some givers prefer to create an aquatic state, close to the immersion in warm water or to the mother's placenta. Using a great deal of oil is frequent in the cocoon style. Others will prefer to use just the necessary quantity in order to prevent the receiver from losing some of the sensitivity which allows a better skin to skin contact between the giver's hands and the receiver's body.

Oiling the body

Either you oil all the parts of the body that you can reach, and with this option you mustn't spare the oil because this will be the only dose the subject will get before you turn them over on their back.

Or else you oil each body part separately before massaging it. This is the method preferred by most givers who find that the energy spreads too fast when they oil the whole body from the start.

Oiling the palms of the hands and the soles of the feet

Either you oil the palms and the soles like the rest of the body, spreading the same oil you poured on the back, the legs and arms, or you refrain from oiling the palms and the soles because this may reduce the subject's sensitivity in these very tactile areas. When you have more experience you will be able to choose which of these approaches suits you best, you and your partner.

The oil-bottle and oil temperature

Prepare the oil in a pouring bottle and place it near the receiver's body so you will always have it to hand. Ideally, you should have a feeding bottle warmer as heat will fluidify your oil and raise it to skin temperature. Otherwise, warm it in a double-boiler if the room temperature is low.

PERSONAL PREPARATION OF THE RECEIVER

Be present. Breathe through the nose, if possible in synch with the person massaging you. Focus on your ventral breathing: inhale and exhale to and from the lower part of your abdomen. Relaxation comes when you exhale, evacuating the thoughts and toxins from your body and mind. The attention you pay to your breathing prevents your thoughts from going round and round in your head. Soon, you will not be thinking of anything. Your letting-go and your confidence will help you to breathe better, to go deeper into yourself and at the same time make you more buoyant. Concentrate on your breathing to find the proper tempo.

If thoughts are still running through your head or if some vague worry is nagging at you, shift immediately your attention to your breathing.

Confidence is essential. Abandon yourself utterly to the man or woman massaging you. The more you relax, the more beneficial the massage will be. Confidence and letting-go will help you go further.

Be neutral and have no expectations: you are a mere witness to what is going on, a witness of your sensations.

Your breath work will diffuse your vital energy to your whole body and different organs, so don't forget to breathe properly.

Letting your sensations overcome you will prompt you to slow down, then your awareness of the moment will open your heart to your surroundings.

The level of awareness characteristic of the Tantra constitutes a third presence co-created by the two partners in the massage.

The golden rules for the receiver:

- Don't plan a massage right after a meal.
- Take a hot shower before the massage. A hot shower is also important before getting dressed again. If you are at home, let the massage soak in first, as a shower might spoil your meditative state. Prolong your pleasure by staying on your back.
- Before the massage begins, tell the other person about your taboos and your no-goes (your particular forms of modesty or sensibility, positions you don't like), or the after-effects of some illness or accident you may have had.
- Spend a moment collecting your thoughts, alone or with the giver.
- Remove all your clothes before lying down.
- Close your eyes.
- The small talk has a negative effect on the massage: only silence can allow for meditation. If you have difficulty emptying your mind, concentrate on what you feel or on the hands of the person massaging you.
- Avoid projecting any affect or sexual desire as they would interfere with the other person's concentration and mar this sacred moment.
- Remember to breathe slowly and deeply through the nose at all times, filling your belly when you inhale, emptying it before you exhale.
- Such a journey requires both of you to be present, so make sure you are present.

Whether you are giving or receiving the massage, a certain detachment is necessary throughout: when we are massaged we content ourselves with existing here and now, with giving love when we massage, bereft of any particular intentionality.

PREPARATION OF THE GIVER

Get at least one massage before you begin massaging other people. Being a receiver will give you a sense of the special form of communication through touching, of the gift that is provided by Tantric massage and the beneficial effects of this gift.

Trying several massages from different partners will give you an idea of the proper touch, the slowness and breadth of the movements, the depth of the relaxation obtained through the contact of the hands during a pause.

Tantra workshops are numerous and trendy these days, and among them are massage workshops, which provide a wide variety of experimentation as you will change partners and roles frequently.

Don't forget you are taking part in a ritual. Everything to do with the Tantra is simultaneously physical and spiritual. Massaging is giving something to the Other, but it is also developing a form of receptiveness which you would not perhaps otherwise possess.

While being attentive to ourselves tends to lead to self-coddling, being attentive to others makes us good listeners, an art difficult to learn which the laying on of hands in a Tantric massage facilitates. (See **Chapter 10**: Specific Tantric massage techniques). Your attentiveness passes entirely through your hands.

Practice the massage with no particular intention, and especially with no intention of surpassing yourself or doing the other person good, though this should not prevent you from improving the quality of your presence and attention. It all happens here and now.

The golden rules for the giver:

- Your nails are short and filed perfectly smooth. Wash your hands before you begin. If they are cold, rinse them in hot water first.
- At the start, ask your partner if your gestures and the pressure you apply feel pleasant. After that, respect the principle of silence during the massage.
- The oil bottle must always be within your grasp, near the thighs or the legs of the subject or near your thigh, to avoid knocking it over and interrupting the contact.
- Make sure you are at a proper distance from the subject to avoid bending your forearms, as bending the elbows takes energy away from your hands.
- Remember to breathe during the massage, to keep your back and neck straight, and to stretch them from time to time to keep your energy and avoid stiffness.
- Your fingers must apply the same degree of pressure as the palm of your hand.
- Avoid rubbing the skin as if you were applying a body lotion.
- Your effleurages (yin touch) must never resemble a caress.
- Press down on the back of the prone receiver at the moment of exhalation.
- Avoid pressing down with all your weight, except for certain stretching effects.
- Let your hands slide easily over the skin, as in a Hawaiian massage which imitates the waves of the ocean, and they should also slip easily under the body thanks to the oil.
- At the end of a move, always remember to bring your hand back towards you.
- Remember to slow down your arm movements and insert pauses.
- Ideally, the breathing from your belly should be synched with your partner's breathing: try to adopt the same rhythm.

- If there should occur a blockage in the person you are massaging, repeat your last gestures. Any stiffness requires a gradual loosening of the contraction.
- Be attentive: if the person moves an arm or a leg, it's because a pressure point has been touched. Repeat the movement, asking whether there is pain in that particular spot.
- Take note of the little resistances that a person's mind generates, resistances in the muscles, the mucous membranes or, on the contrary the little abandonments, when the areas you are massaging grow softer, and accompany them.
- When you have had enough experience to have the proper gestures, concentrate on your hands rather than on the techniques. The receiver must feel a presence in your hands.
- Be totally in the present, without thinking of anything and especially without wondering "am I doing this person good?"
- If a male subject has an erection, it is not an invitation but merely a frequent reaction of his libido. Remain neutral.

THE FLEXIBILITY OF THE GIVER

To be able to give a traditional Tantric massage it is best to warm up. Massaging on the floor can be hard on the neck, the back, the pelvis and the arms if you are out of training or stiff. After a while, some people's thighs hurt, with others it is the knees. They'll prefer to change positions. By crouching or sitting on the floor at some stage in the massage or using a low prayer stool, for example.

Stretching, dancing and Yoga are activities which loosen up the back and pelvis in ways very appropriate to massaging on the floor. Here are three exercises to help you reach all the parts of the subject's body without aching.

- Sit with your legs stretched out in front of you. Try to touch your toes with your finger-tips and keep this position for two or three minutes: this will limber up the small of your back.
- Stand with your legs apart to the width of your hips, drop your head forward to knee-level. Straighten up in slow motion, lifting your head when your back is straight. Do several round of this.
- As in every type of massage, your fingers are also called into play, even though this type mainly involves the whole palm. Think of a pianist. Loosen up those little joints by pressing and then stretching them. Stretch your fingers. Push them back with the other hand.

CHAPTER 9

CONNECTING
WITH YOUR PARTNER

After the hot shower which functions as an airlock between your previous situation and the massage itself, the partners sit facing one another the time to collect their thoughts in silence. If the receiver is a beginner, then the giver can be the guide and use the appropriate words to generate the right mood. If you and your partner are both Tantrikas, the ritual bow will help to open the heart and to see what is divine in your partner.

GUIDING THE RECEIVER

➤ While sitting cross-legged face to face, the giver may give their partner instructions: "close your eyes, let your thoughts run through your mind like clouds in the sky without dwelling on any of them, let your shoulders droop..."

➤ Put your partner in touch with their body and their sensations, noticing the coolness of the air inhaled, the warmth of the air exhaled. Place a verbal emphasis on the deep breathing with an open mouth which should be maintained throughout the massage.

THE RITUAL BOW

- In the same position, join hands at heart-level looking into each other's eyes for a few minutes to establish the connection.
- Point your hands at the floor in order to draw the energy from the earth while taking a long deep breath.
- When you breathe out, lean forward until your forehead touches your partner's.
- Join hands again over your heart as you breathe in, point them down breathing out.

The heart is at the center of the Tantra because of all the love that the givers put into their hands and the opening that allows their partner to receive it.

THE WHO-AM-I?

This is an alternative to the ritual bow, especially when the partners do not know each other. The exercise is described in **chapter** 7. After collecting your thoughts with your eyes closed which will settle your minds, the partners gaze straight into one another's eyes for several minutes. This eye-contact intimacy generates discomfort. The exercise places you at the centre of yourself, connected to the Other and in the present moment, rid of all your social layers and daily problems. In some cases it enables you to distance yourselves from sexual expectations.

THE TIBETAN BOWL

The sound and the reverberations of a Tibetan bowl combined with the diffusion of an essential oil meant to develop the aura allow us to raise our level of spirituality and get into the right mood for the massage. They help our energy's transformation. The surprising thing is the degree to which a good Tibetan bowl (the best ones are cast at full moon time) is receptive to the blockages a person may have in one or another area of their body: a singing bowl falls silent on an area where the energy circulates badly or not at all, but continues to sing on the rest of a prone body. When a professional masseuse treats a stranger, she will often prefer to undertake a little energy cleansing with a Tibetan bowl by ringing it between the subject and herself after the initial meditation, in particular when she senses, through the energy he gives out, that he has sexual expectations.

CHAPTER 10

THE TANTRIC MASSAGE

The Tantric massage rebuilds the energy consumed by tensions, allowing us to discover the original strength within us through the therapeutic power of sensual pleasure. The tempo is slow: the idea being to slow down your natural city tempo and guide you to a greater inwardness, awaken your energy and make it circulate, bring to life every cell of your body. This journey of self-discovery allows us to be in tune with ourselves. Its effects last approximately three days.

NUDITY AND LETTING GO

Barring a reluctance on the part of one of the partners which they will have discussed beforehand, the giver will wear some piece of underwear (nakedness is an option if a couple is involved, though it can get out of hand), while the receiver of the massage is naked. If they feel embarrassed about shedding all their clothes, a disposable piece of underwear may be worn.

A Tantric massage is the most sensual of all massages without being sexual so just let yourself go. Accept the over-all nature of the massage, have no special expectations. In these moments, your genitals are on a par with the other parts of your body and

yet are not the object of any special attention or insistence in the course of such a massage: they are rubbed, touched lightly or avoided in accordance with your desire or your degree of Tantra.

SPECIFIC TANTRIC MASSAGE TECHNIQUES

LAYING ON OF HANDS

A Tantric massage is punctuated or terminated by resting the hands on two remote chakras. These pauses are often described as a "laying on of hands", term borrowed from certain religious or healing practices, but their function should not be confused with the latter. These pauses between taking care of two areas calm the body and the mind. The motionless hands of the giver set up a current of energy which links earth to sky through the body and mind of the receiver. The chakras, in the shape of a funnel with the wide end pointing towards the back, open up little by little

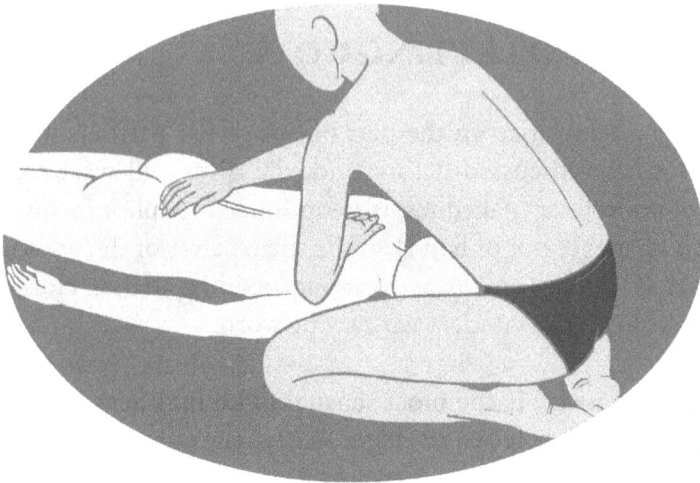

Figure 5. Laying on of hands.

to the current connecting them. Pausing on specific body points confers a meditative quality to the massage: we move into the mind via the body.

INTEGRATION

This is the name given to the globalizing phase: we extend the energy produced by the laying on of hands and localized massage to the entire lower or upper body with long sliding strokes. In the integration phase we apply an even pressure with the whole hand, fingers pressed together. This is the firm touch, the yang. For a yin, practice by raking the fingertips, spread claw-like, from top to bottom. Go up gently, and back down again slowly. The yin touch draws the sensitivity out of the dermis and nerve-endings to the surface of the skin. It awakens the receiver's sensibility and sensuality. Practice slowness: allow for example 10 seconds for a two-handed sliding move down the spinal column. At the end of this globalization, take a pause with one hand on the sacrum, the other on the back over the heart chakra. If you are tall enough, link the heart to the perinea with this laying on of hands.

THE DIFFERENT STYLES OF TANTRIC MASSAGE

A beginner will find it hard to adopt any particular style at first: you will be too engrossed with the changes of your position, the movements of your hands and the management of the oil. However once you have carved out a path for yourself around the receiver's body you can develop a massage style of you own since your mind will be less burdened by learning the basic steps. Your style may vary according to your mood or the expectations of the receiver. You may quickly adopt a yang touch or a yin touch according to their expectations, or you can alternate them (see Chapter 6). Each style lays greater emphasis on one of the four bodies, the mental, the physical, the emotional or the spiritual body.

We distinguish between:

- The meditative massage is ruled by slowness and inwardness and is mainly addressed to the spiritual body but does not exclude sensual delight.
- The emotional massage takes us to the deepest level of our being, brings out emotions, tears and laughter, which can appear before the massage but also afterwards.
- The cocoon style massage combines the two previous styles with the addition of mothering intentions or gestures.
- The energetic massage actually uses the receiver's sexual energy to augment their overall energy.

WHICH MASSAGE TO CHOOSE?

There are practically as many types of Tantric massages as there are masseurs/euses. How much sharing are you prepared to accept? Do you have special problems? It might be anorgasmia, premature ejaculation, frigidity, lack of sexual desire, or you may simply be out of step with reality, out of step with the Other, in a permanent state of stress, have an attention deficit disorder, suffer from a lack of self-respect, epidermal numbness or just feel awful all the time. Before you settle on your massage style, try two or three different kinds corresponding to the various styles on offer. Your sensations will lead to broadening the pallet of your experience.

TANTRIC MASSAGES BY SELF-EMPLOYED PROFESSIONALS

It is important to find a good professional. With a masseur/euse who comes to your home, you must look upon the massage as a ritual. It will be preceded by a face to face meditation. It is a total massage, including the genitals. A total massage makes it possible to go beyond sex despite the nudity, which is often synonymous with sexual availability in the mind of an outsider.

What should one ask over the phone?

If you are considering an individual proposition from a masseur/euse discovered on the Internet or by word of mouth, there is nothing to prevent you from checking them out.

Ring them up and ask the questions that will enlighten you:

- How long do they give you to relax after the massage?
- What other forms of massage did they practice before changing to Tantric massage?
- Do they work on the floor (which is more authentic and allows for true sharing) or on a table?
- Do they have some kind of heater (in the event the massage is taking place in winter)?
- If you don't like the idea of keeping the oil on your body after the massage, is a shower available?

Kashmiri massages

These combine cradling and embracing. They concern areas of sensibility and emotions that are different from those of a Tantric massage. There are fewer professionals offering these, and they are often quite expensive because of the intimacy involved. For this reason, a masseuse may refuse to give this type of massage to someone who has never had one, even though a piece of underwear does separate their two bodies: a beginner may misinterpret the bodies' proximity. The intimacy of this form of massage is such that the prodigious sharing it procures must be reserved for people who already have notions of the Tantra.

Therapeutic Tantric massages

These are meant for anyone who has a blockage of the first chakra, they treat libido problems, and particularly people who encounter difficulties being aroused or reaching orgasm.

They make it possible to open the path to sexual energy through the re-appropriation of a person's genitals. A person with a weak libido will discover unknown emotions and sensations, others achieve a better mechanical reactivity of their genitals, thanks to karsei nei tsang, for example, that ancient Chinese massage which tones up the circulation in the lower parts of our body (see Chapter 18).

Sexual Tantric massages

Within a couple, it is frequent to reach one or more orgasms through the direct manipulation of the penis or the vagina, the man's testicles or the woman's labia, majora and minora. Sexual massages are rarely Tantric, strictly speaking: rather, they are erotic massages. They have been called "Tantric" because the term is fashionable. Tantric sexual stimulation is dealt with in the last chapter.

The massage of the genitals takes place within the framework of an overall Tantric massage when the partners are Tantrikas. The genitals are massaged just like the rest of the body.

CHAPTER 11

THE TANTRIC MASSAGE
FOR BEGINNERS

Duration: 90 minutes

This type of massage enables you to move around the receiver by sliding on the cloth all around their body. You can focus on the zones you massage and be close enough to get the right move, your hand flat on the receiver's skin and your fingers together. You don't have to stretch to reach certain parts, or lean on the person's body. Your strokes are not as sweeping as in the traditional Tantric massage because you are not working in the axis of the kundalinî (head to feet) but they are more detailed and precise.

A short giver who has to deal with a tall receiver may encounter limits. It will be difficult to reach the torso from the feet and vice versa. Indeed, the long sliding moves of the traditional Tantric massage as described below take place along a single axis, from head to feet. If your heights are very different (or if your back lacks flexibility) choose the star-shaped massage. You will glean other techniques from traditional Tantric massage in **chapter 12** when you have made some progress.

The receiver is naked. As a giver you wear some undergarment in order not to be distracted or to distract the subject from the meditative and emotional side of a Tantric massage.

THE STAR-SHAPED POSITIONS OF THE GIVER

These positions correspond to the five points of a star around the receiver's body. You slide around your partner on your knees. This way you will always be close to the area you are working on. Back away or move closer to find the appropriate distance. If sitting on your heels is tiring your thighs or your knees, you may sit on the floor, while massaging the feet or the face for example. Some professional masseuses use a small prayer stool that they move around the receiver. It is important to be in such a position as to keep your arms straight, except when massaging certain areas (upper back, torso) with your forearms. It takes a bit of practice to learn how to synchronize the different phases of the massage when sliding from one position to the next.

— The giver is sitting on their heels with spread knees behind the subject's head. Place your hands on the heart chakra and leave them there in silence from 10 to 20 seconds and meanwhile, try to synchronize your breathing with your partner's.

OILING

— Pour a small quantity of oil into your cupped hands rather than directly onto the subject's skin. If you do not have a baby-bottle warmer to take the chill off the oil, rub it between your palms.
— Moisten the back and the inside of the arms down to the back of the hands. You needn't use a great deal of oil, the important thing is for your hands to slide smoothly.

MASSAGING THE UPPER BACK AND SHOULDERS

—➤ Join your two hands at neck-level. Be careful to keep your arms straight.

—➤ Use long strokes all the way down to the small of the back and buttocks with both hands, symmetrically or asymmetrically, to spread the oil. The first stage of a Tantric massage is meant to relax the receiver; a tense person is not sufficiently in touch with their body.

—➤ Knead the trapezoids and the shoulders. With your thumbs, press on the tissues, but without digging in: this is neither shiatsu nor a Thai massage.

—➤ Alternate this kneading of the muscles with long sliding moves over the back, but also on the subject's sides so that they will feel enveloped. Repeat this until you feel the area becoming limber.

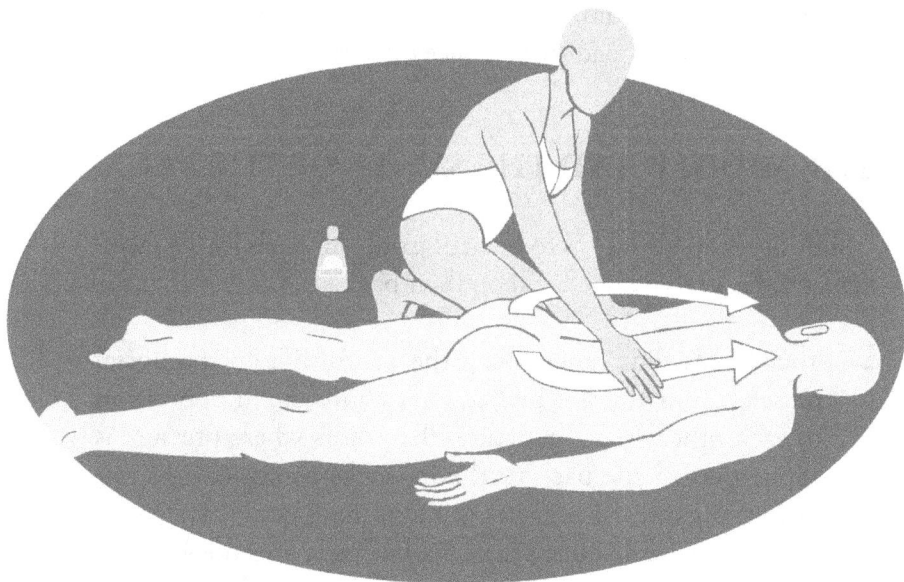

Figure 6. Oiling and massaging the upper back and shoulders.

- You may also lean forward and massage the back with your forearms, elbows bent.
- Make smaller and smaller circles on either side of the spinal column with your hands turned outwards in order to dispel tension.
- Five points between the shoulder blades correspond to the the heart chakra and may be massaged gently in tiny circles with the tips of two or three fingers.

In order to rid an area of tension, your hand-movements are counter-clockwise.

- The edges of both hands slide symmetrically down the spinal column without too much pressure, then up and down a few times. This repeated move stimulates the neuro-vegetative system.
- Finish with a laying on of hands, one on the heart and the other on the sacrum.
- Integrate with broad strokes. (see Integration in **Chapter 10**)

THE MIDDLE AND THE SMALL OF THE BACK

Slide over the cloth so as to be sitting on your heels by the receiver's thighs, keeping one hand on their back.

- Your hands slide down along the axis of life on the dorsal muscles. Your thumbs lie flat, your hands are in opposition to each other. In acupuncture, the points where pressure is applied down the back to the buttocks correspond to our various organs: the lungs at the top, the digestive system in the middle, while points near the bottom correspond to our circulation, kidneys, intestines and adrenal glands which manage our anxiety levels.

- With your whole hand repeat the sliding moves down both sides of the spine, and then up.
- Pull yourself up on your knees and stretch the subject's back by pushing down a bit with outstretched arms. Repeat this stretching.
- Do it again placing your hands diagonally, which will enable you to stretch the back side-wise.
- Take a 10 seconds pause, keeping one hand on the sacrum, the other above the nape of the neck, thus connecting the lower and upper chakras.
- Integrate.

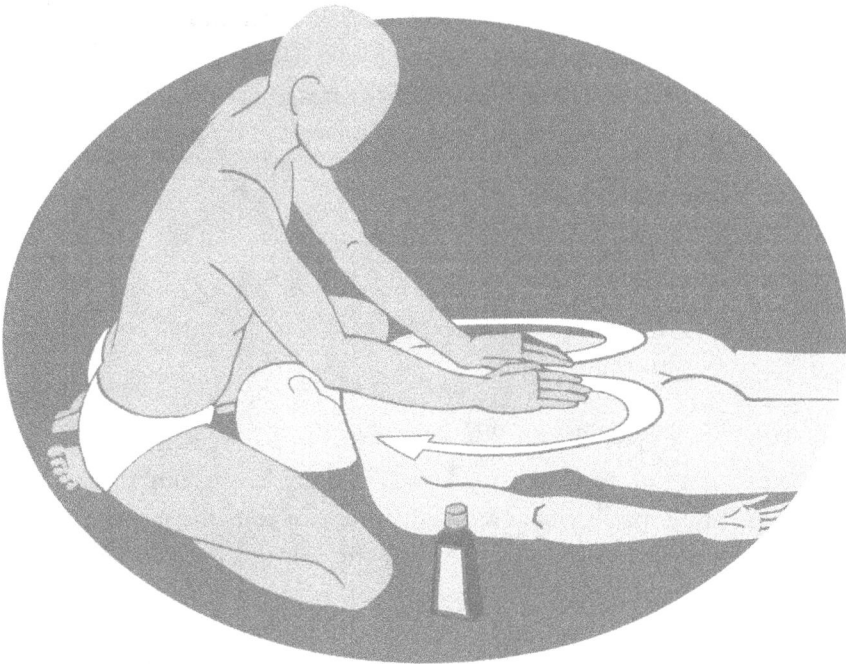

Figure 7. The middle and the small of the back.

HIPS, THIGHS AND SACRUM

- Squat close to the body. Run your hands over their hips, knead the buttocks, massage the thighs with the whole of both hands, applying the same pressure with the palms and fingers. Work from the outside to the inside, then from top to bottom and vice versa. The movement ends in the small of the back with your hands turned out.
- Wrap the lower part of the back in your two hands and slide slowly towards the receiver's sides. Repeat this reassuring wrapping movement two or three times.
- Next massage in little circles the two lateral points located at the top of the sacrum: they facilitate the evacuation of toxins and have a direct action on the bladder. Don't be afraid to press hard on these two points with your thumbs, keeping your arms straight.
- Take a pause, with one hand over the heart, the other on the sacrum to connect the chakras and provoke a flow of energy.
- Integrate with sliding pressures on either side of the spine.

FEET

Slide back a bit on the cloth.

- When you have found the ideal position for massaging the feet, take one foot in your hands and lay it on your thigh. You should be sitting at an angle so as not to turn your back on the receiver. Massage the sole, the sides of the foot, and the toes.
- Slide on your behind to change your position slightly to the other side or order to massage the other foot. (See description and illustration of foot massage **Chapter 7**).

Variant:

— Straddling one or both of your partner's legs.
— For this stage of the massage, you may step over the receiver's thigh so that your knees are on both sides of one leg, or else you may straddle both thighs.
— Resume the long strokes up and down their back.

FIST ON THE PERINEUM

— While kneeling between the receiver's legs, you may finish this part of the massage pressing the perineum with your fist. Push firmly upwards and maintain the pressure for from 10 to 20 seconds in order to awaken the sexual energy stored in this area.
— You may finish massaging the back with a yin touch: brushing your hand lightly over the skin.

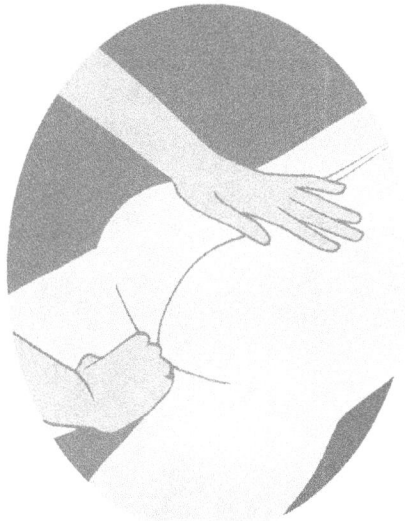

Figure 8. Fist on the perineum.

ABDOMEN

Slide over the cloth so that you are sitting on your heels near the person's hips. As their genitals are exposed, the receiver will feel vulnerable. Your first moves will be designed to allay apprehensions, conscious or unconscious.

>— Rock the abdomen from side to side with both hands together, then massage it clockwise, one hand resting on the other without exerting pressure, then one hand behind the other.
>— Finish with a pause, hands superposed over the dantian.
>— Now slide one hand up to the receiver's torso before changing position without breaking the contact.

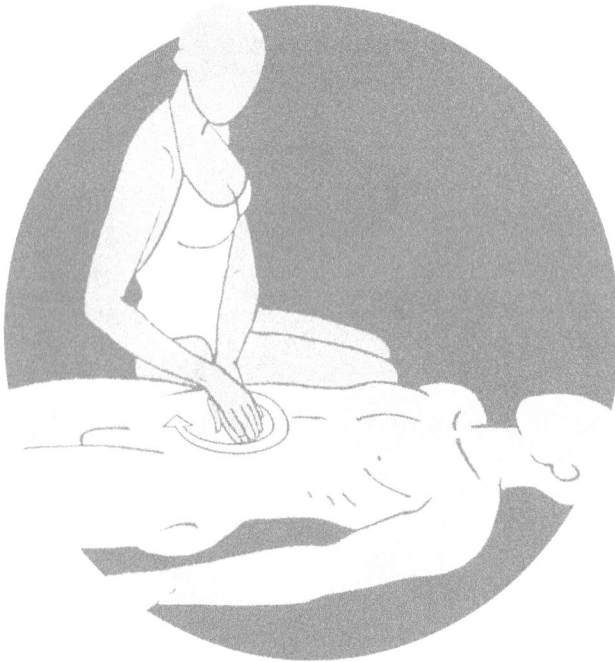

Figure 9. Massaging the belly.

ARMS AND HANDS

Slide a few inches towards the upper body to be near the receiver's arm.

- Wrap both hands around the shoulder in a sliding move down the arm all the way to the wrist. If the back is well oiled, you shouldn't need to add more. Otherwise, pour a bit on the shoulder while keeping one hand in contact with the skin.
- Knead the arm from shoulder to elbow, then apply slow sliding pressure.
  Repeat the movement from shoulder to wrist with both hands.
- Slide to the middle of the palm and press the hollow with both thumbs, then knead the fingers one at a time.
- Take a 10 to 20 seconds pause keeping one hand on the wrist, the other over the heart.

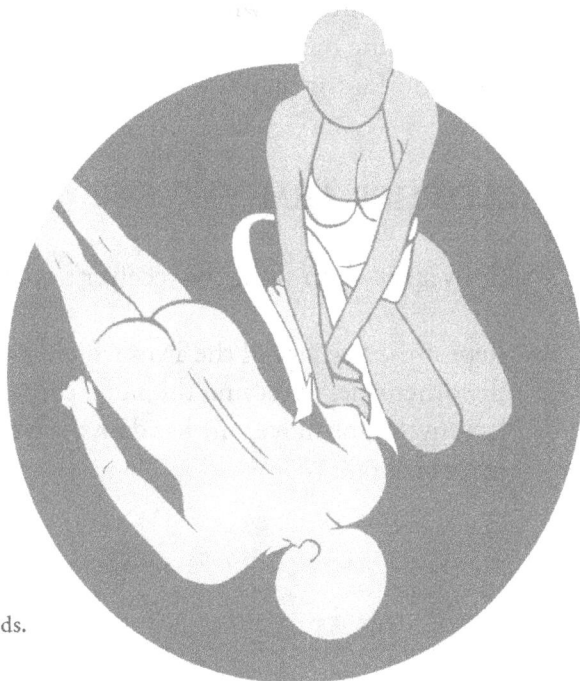

Figure 10. Arms and hands.

LEGS AND GENITALS (OPTIONAL)

Slide over the cloth to your partner's feet and sit between the legs in order to give your thighs and knees a bit of a rest. While you are moving, keep one hand on the receiver's thigh then slide it down to their ankle.

- Massage the legs from bottom to top on the inner face, one hand following the other.
- If you are about to massage the genitals (lingam or yoni) slide between the subject's legs in order to place your forearm in such a way that it is neither too far from the perineum nor too close to it (see Massage of the genitals, **Chapter 16**).
- Delicately massage the crotch and the inner face of the thighs with a yin touch.

However, we generally do not massage the genitals during a first massage. You and your partner must be sufficiently experienced to avoid any confusion with a sexual massage which would be prejudicial to the meditative, emotional and energetic effects of the authentic Tantric massage.

THE OTHER ARM

Slide over the cloth along the receiver's other side to the torso.

- Repeat the massage of the arms which you have just done on the other side, observing the same pause which ended your last enveloping move, one hand on the wrist, the other on the heart chakra.

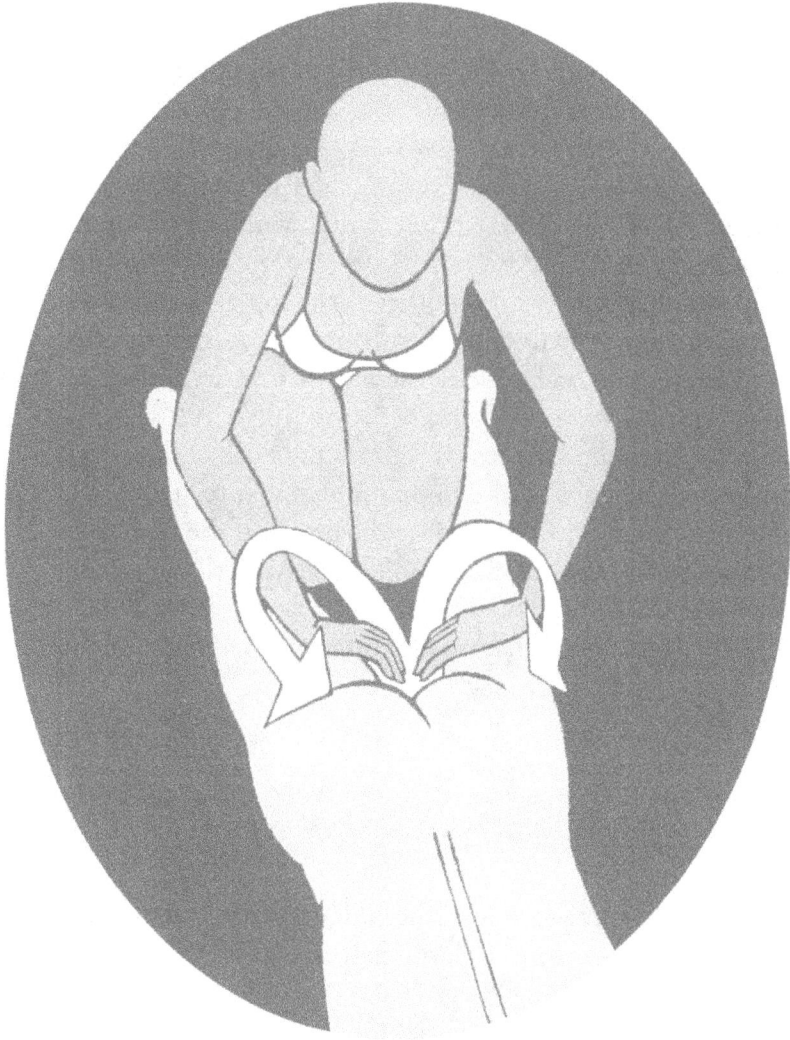

Figure 11. Legs and genitals.

CHEST

Slide over the cloth and place your knees behind your subject's head keeping the contact with one hand.

- Gently press the shoulders towards the feet then slide your hands towards the center of the sternum with an enveloping movement.
- Cup your hands over one another at the top of the sternum for a moment, then slide them downwards side by side between the pectoral muscles, moving them apart at the base of the ribs.
- At waist level, slip your hands beneath the small of their back and take a pause. Pull the body towards you to stretch the lower back and possibly massage the breasts if the receiver is female, or the pectoral muscles of a male, with slow, rotating movements.
- Apply a laying on of hands, one on the solar plexus or the heart, the other on the navel.
- Integrate.

FACE

Move your knees forward on either side of the receiver's head. For this last stage of the massage you may also sit on the floor.

- You may wish to massage the face for 10 minutes, as described in Chapter 7 "Korean face massage".
- You will finish by resting your hands on your partner's eyelids or temples in order to dispel any sense of abandonment or loneliness which may come over them if there is a loss of contact between you.

You will wait until they open their eyes and discover you sitting over them, before moving away.

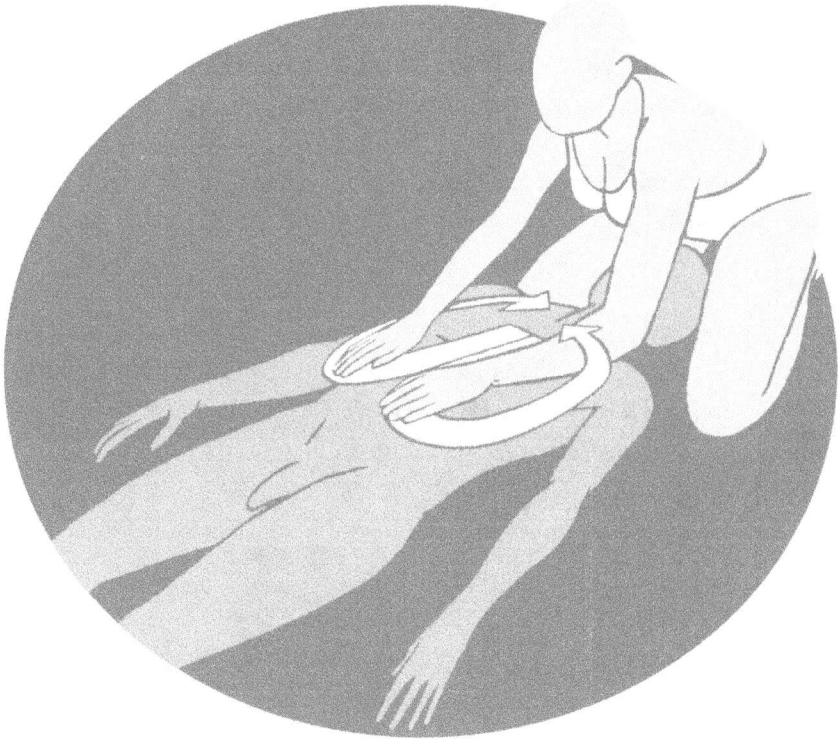

Figure 12. Chest.

ENDING THE MASSAGE

Be careful not to withdraw your hands too quickly. You may choose between:

- A ying touch on the arms and torso.
- A slow sweeping movement over the whole body with a silky fabric or a soft, warm towel (yin).
- Laying on of hands over the 7th and 6th chakras (at the top of the skull and the middle of the forehead: they are called the "crown" and the "third eye").
- A laying on of hands over the closed eyelids. (See figure 21 at the end of **Chapter 12**).

> ### My advice
> *When you have done two or three star-shaped massages, go to the next chapter to glean a few new tips and moves from traditional Tantric massage.*

CHAPTER 12

TRADITIONAL
TANTRIC MASSAGE

Duration: 90 to 120 minutes

Pulling the receiver's hands over their head and lay your palms on theirs. Take a short pause then bring them to their heart. Now slowly withdraw your hands.

- Kneeling or squatting on the cloth behind the receiver's head, lay a firm hand on their neck and the other on their sacrum. This is the first laying on of hands.
- After 10-15 seconds, move the hand that has been resting on the neck down the back with a sliding pressure until it meets the hand resting on the sacrum. Take another pause with your hands next to each other or the one lying on the other. If words are to be spoken during the massage, it is now that you should speak, before the partner has entered into an altered state of awareness resembling a meditation. You can remind them of the need to inhale with the belly and exhale through the mouth, that deep breathing through the mouth allows the energy from the massage to spread to the whole body.
To help them relax, you can repeat that there is nothing to desire, nothing to wish for, nothing to expect throughout the massage. Or you can demand absolute silence during the

massage, allowing both partners to focus all their attention, the one on their gift of energy and love through the hands, the other on their body in the present moment, the here and now.

The massage will increase the subject's presence to their body and emotions, their mind and spiritual being.

OILING

Placing your partner's head between your thighs, keep one hand in contact with their body and with the other pour a small amount of warm oil (for lack of a warmer, warm it with your palms) on the receiver's back. Spread it all over the back, the sides, the shoulders and arms, applying the same, even pressure with the whole hand, fingers joined.

MASSAGING THE SIDES, BACK, SHOULDERS, AND BUTTOCKS

— While oiling, make it a point of loosening up the receiver.
— Use the pincer technique (pinching the skin) to unwind the tensions in the neck and trapezoid muscles, if necessary.
— Knead them like bread-dough but do not linger.
— Put pressure on the middle of the back to empty the subject's lungs and force them to breathe in deeply.
— Your oiled palms slide down over the ribs, oiling the subject's sides. You may also slide both palms under their sides and move upwards in a two-handed enveloping movement.
— Do at least three rounds of these moves with the same pressure on each region. Slide your hands slowly all the way down the arms. Next, with fingers fanned out, your hands slide in broad symmetrical patterns towards the hollow of the back, then towards the edges.

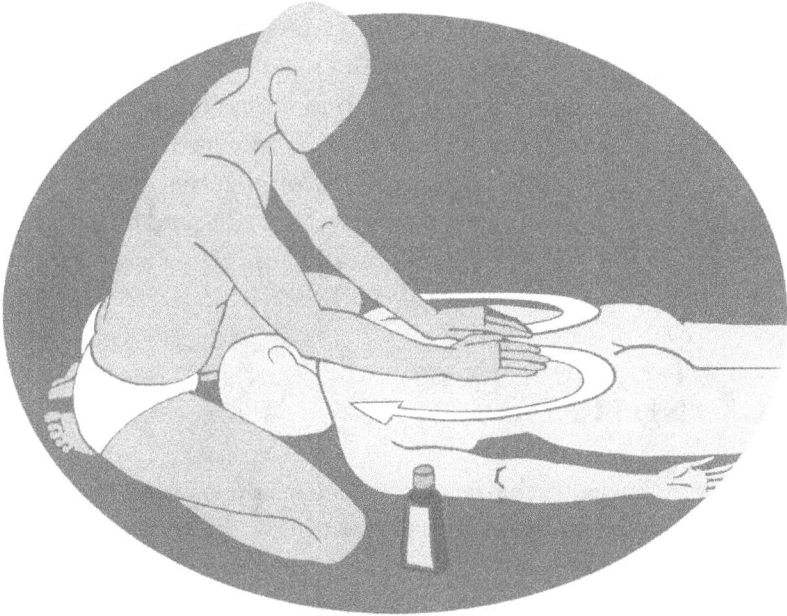

Figure 13. Oiling the body.

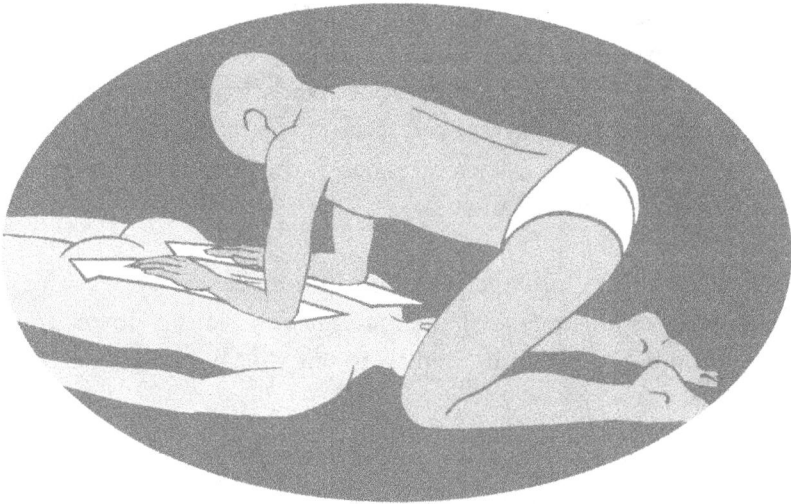

Figure 14. Sides, back, shoulders, and buttocks.

- You may alternate these sliding moves across the back with kneading the shoulders. Use your forearms for these slow sliding movements: this is the only occasion when your elbows are bent. The rest of the time, your arms are straight.
- Lean over your subject to spread the oil that may have been absorbed into the upper back to the lower back and buttocks. To reach the buttocks, draw yourself up on your knees if need be.

LEGS AND FEET

Slide your knees to the receiver's feet keeping your hand on their back while you move around their body. Sit on your heels. With your free hand, bring the oil-bottle closer. Be careful to place yourself in line with their head and feet, the Kundalinî axis. Keep one hand on the receiver's back while you pour more oil on it, if necessary.

- Oil the backs of the thighs and legs with long symmetrical movements down to the feet.
- Now move up again, sliding your hands from the outside under the legs as far as you can reach.
- Massage several times with both hands the outside of the legs and thighs symmetrically.

Back away on the cloth and grasp one of the receiver's feet with both hands. For this phase of the massage you may sit down to give your joints a rest. You are slightly to one side, but still close to the head-feet axis.

TANTRIC AND KASHMIRI MASSAGES

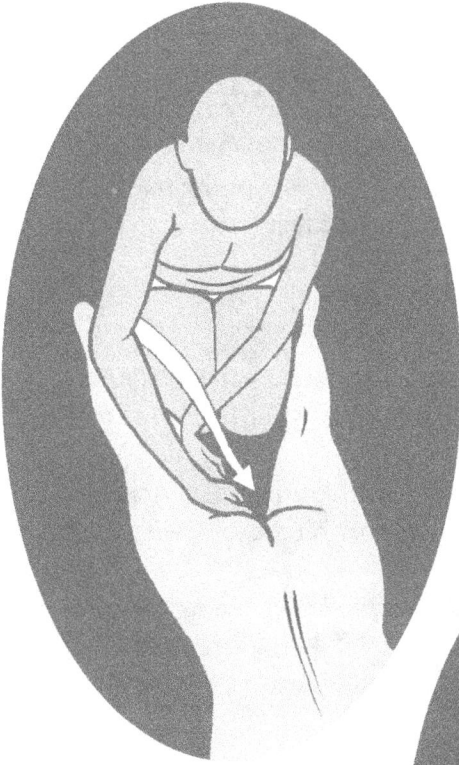

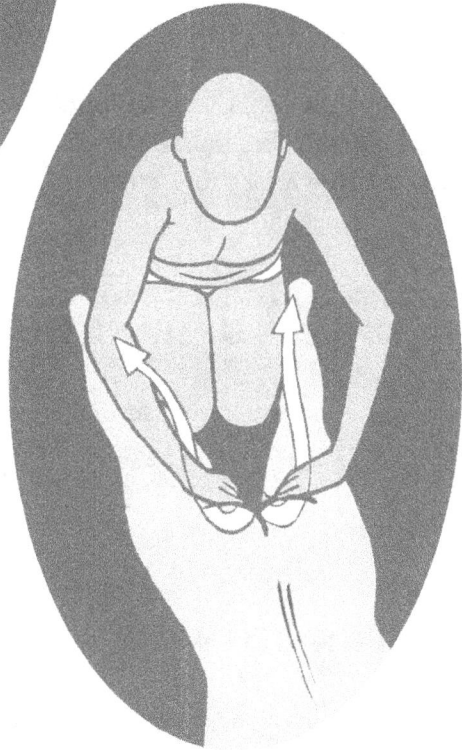

Figures 15.-16. Legs and feet.

- Begin by working on the hollow located just behind the ball of the foot at the base of the big toe, a third of the way along the sole towards the heel. If need be, you may bend the receiver's leg. The foot chakra is important: it is what earths us. If you wish to spend more time on this part of the massage, refer to the paragraph on massaging the feet (see **Chapter 7**).

Move down again on the outside of the thigh and leg.

- Next comes the arching interior of each leg, up to the sacrum. This corresponds to a meridian. One of your hands follows the other leg.
- Massage the calf, exerting pressure with the heel of your hand.
- Massage all around the knee, then work on the joint with your fingers.
- Next massage the other foot, the other chakra under the sole, before proceeding to the other leg.
- Finish with a pause, cupping your hands over the sacrum for a few seconds.

LAYING ON OF HANDS

One hand rests on the sacrum, the other on the neck. Thanks to the gradual opening of these two chakras, warmed and activated by the pressure of your cupped hands, their energy will irrigate the other chakras. (See **figure 5** in **Chapter 10**).

INTEGRATION

- If you have been sitting on the ground, you kneel again between the receiver's knees and you massage both of them with large symmetrical movements, moving up the outer

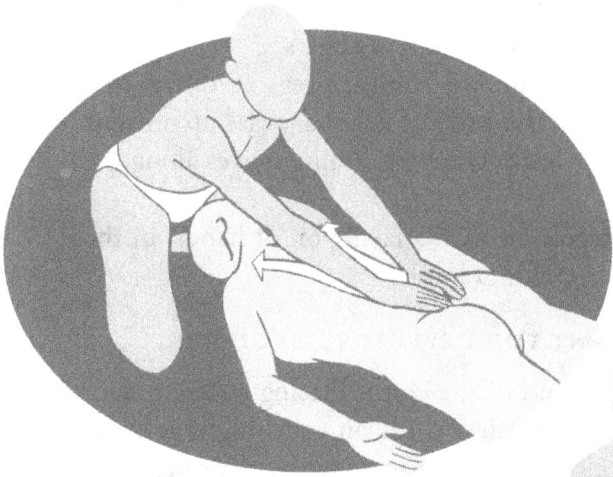

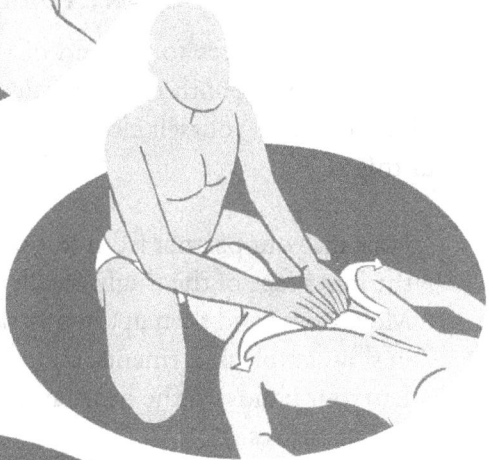

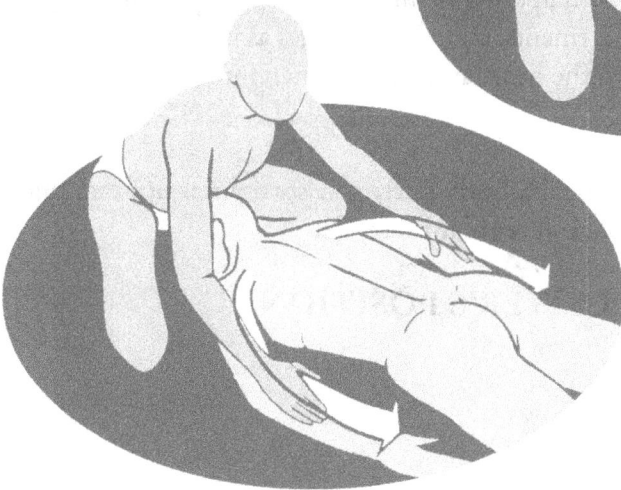

Figures 17. Integration.

surface and down the inner, then vice versa, always applying the same pressure with your palms and joined fingers.

— Move closer, sliding between your subject's legs to diffuse the energy in the lower part of the body: if necessary, rise up on your knees to reach the upper back. Use long sliding moves along the spinal column.

You may conclude this integration with a laying on of hands, in the regions of the heart and sacrum for example.

AN INTEGRATION VARIANT FOR EXPERIENCED GIVERS

Slide on your knees to the end of the cloth. Placing yourself at an angle, you may lay both of the receiver's legs on your thighs at knee-level or else place yourself close to their crotch and lay their pelvis on your thighs.

— Massage your partner from feet to perineum with broad moves on the inner face of the thighs and legs —or else both legs together. Move down and then up, two or three times, then up to the thighs in slow, ample movements, covering the sides as well.

— Lay your hands on the heart and sacrum, then integrate with long sliding moves.

—

After having massaged each body-part, you straighten up, making sure to stretch your back at regular intervals.

CHANGING RECEIVER'S POSITION

Slide on your knees towards the right side of your subject in order to turn them over. Ideally, the receiver should remain in a state of meditative consciousness. Experienced professionals have no problem turning a subject over who is not too massive.

The easiest way to do this is to begin by lifting a leg and an arm, swinging the person three-fourths of the way over before laying them on their back. This is done in stages, massaging the subject at each little move. Here is the way the transition takes place.

Rather than passing directly from a flat on the back to a face down position, a quick transition which may prove difficult, especially if the receiver is heavier than you are, gently push the sole of their left foot upwards with the palm of your left hand so as to bend the left leg at the knee. The bent leg now forms a right angle (90°) on the cloth. This is a sensuous position since the subject's genitals are exposed and they can feel this.

Massage their body with firm sliding moves, the sacrum, then the left arm, then slide upwards.

Dislodge the right arm, which may be trapped beneath the torso. Slide it upwards.

Seize the left leg under the knee, straighten out the leg and gently roll the subject's torso over on the side. The upper back and head will follow the movement.

Add more oil if necessary to massage the left side, then roll the pelvis and extend the right leg completely.

The receiver is now lying on their back. The baring of the receiver's genitals will generate a certain apprehension or anxiety. Consequently, your moves should be very enveloping.

MASSAGING THE LEGS AND BELLY

Slide down to the receiver's feet and in between their legs. Add more

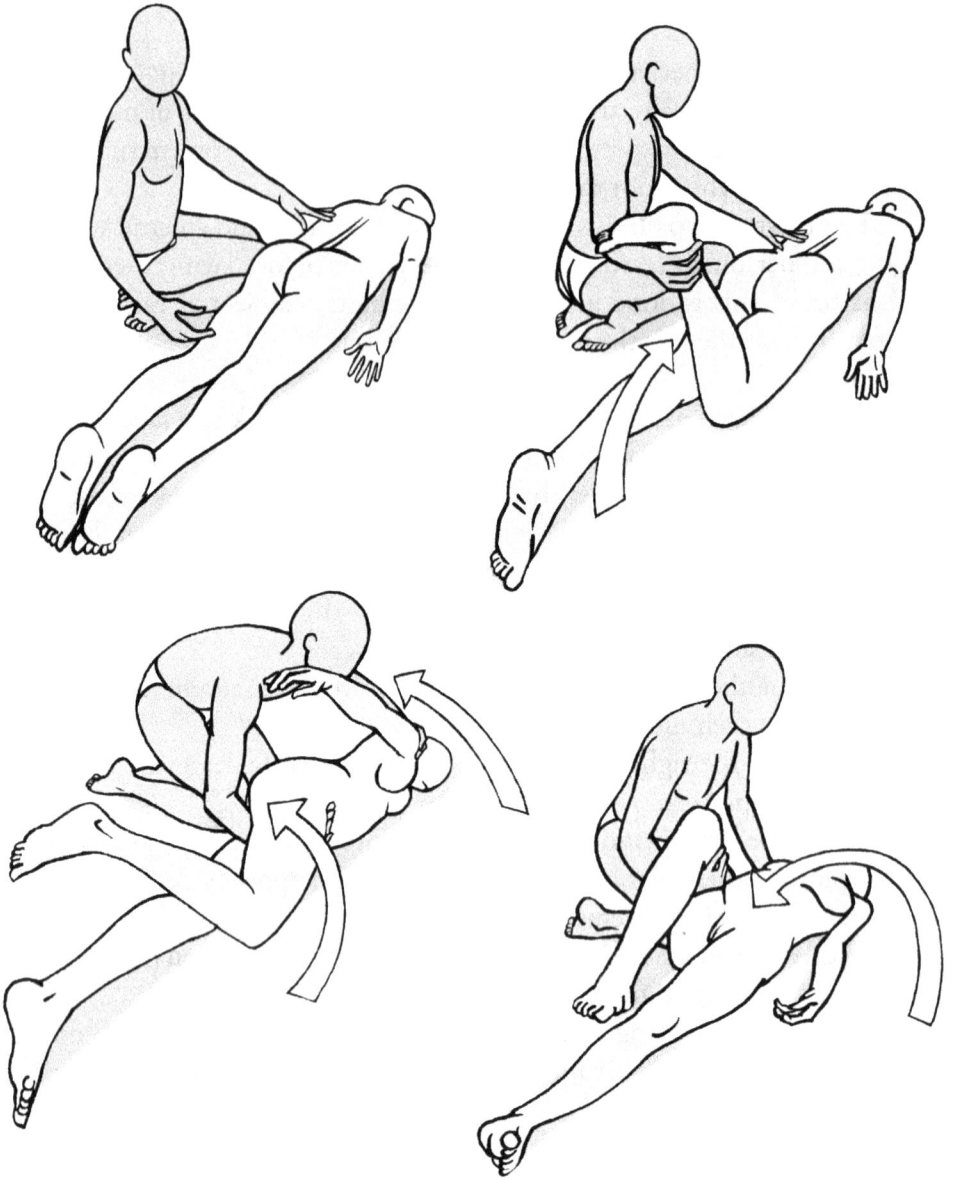

Figure 18 Changing position: Aurélie Sellier's tips.

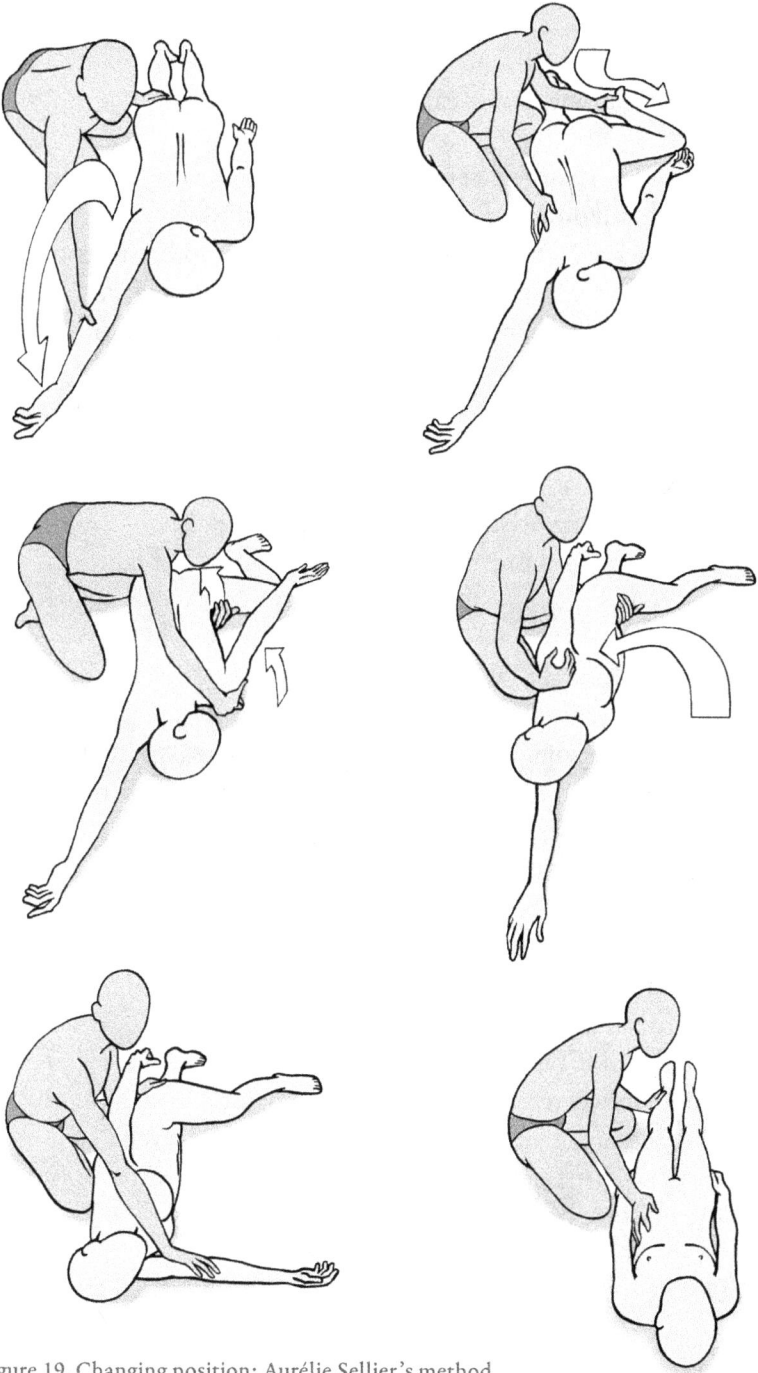

Figure 19. Changing position: Aurélie Sellier's method.

oil if need be, without breaking the contact.

Massage symmetrically the legs up to the crotch then slide one hand down a leg while the other moves up.
Slip between the legs on the cloth to get closer, staying in the same axis. Massage the belly, keeping to the surface.
Rock your partner slowly from one side to the other with both hands, putting all the love you can into it.
Add more oil if required and then move up in sliding circles to the sternum.
Take a pause, one hand on the belly beneath the navel (the dantian), the other cupped over the genitals.
Integrate, and finish with another laying on of hands.

GENITALS

If you are a beginner, delicately massage the groin, the inner face of the thighs, with a ying or yang touch according to the circumstances: a ying touch might be mistaken for a caress.
Take the subject by the sides and lift them slightly, rubbing up and down beneath the ribs and under the thighs.
Take your pause with one fist on the perineum, the other hand flat on the pubis, thus the genital area will be included in the massage.
Premo, the Tantra leader, says: "learning the Tantra is to build a bridge between the genitals and the heart." Massaging the sex organ (lingam, yoni) can be envisaged in the event of a good mastery of Tantric massage as a whole. If you are experienced, go to the massage of the genitals (see **Chapter 16**).

TORSO

If you can't reach the torso, move up between the receiver's

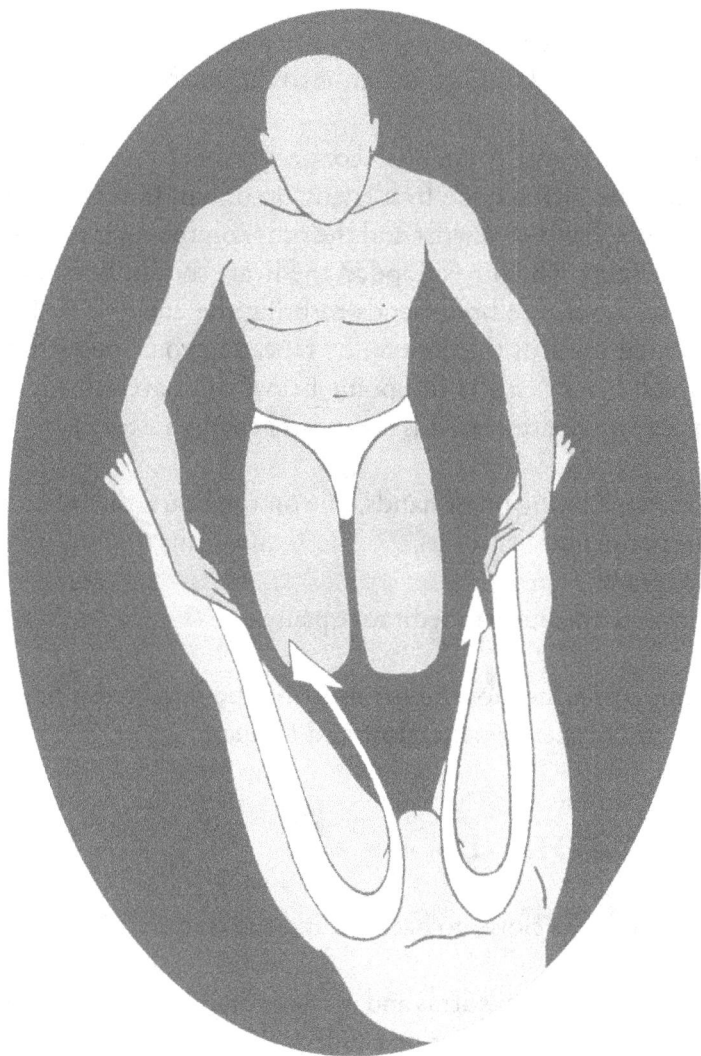

Figure 20. Legs and belly.

thighs.

Massage the torso towards the solar plexus. Add oil if necessary and spread it down the arms to the wrists, one arm after the other.

— You must regularly establish connections between the different parts of the body by a laying on of hands, for example with one hand on a wrist and the other on the solar plexus.

— The energy which has flooded the heart should flow down to the navel: use both hands to bring the energy you have released towards the dantian by repeating your long strokes

— several times: this is the point below the navel where the energy originates, but it is also where energy is stored.

Execute a laying on of hands, one on the heart, the other on the perineum.

Integrate.

— Finish with another meditative pause.

The tempo of your movements must be the same from beginning to end of the massage, slow and regular.

ARMS AND HANDS

Sliding over the cloth, go back behind the receiver's head.

Spread the person's arms and massage their inner sides several times, with sliding motions and/or successive pressures with the heel of your hand all the way down the arms.

— Massage the hands and the hollow of the palms with a slow revolving motion of one or two fingertips, stretching each phalanx and pinching the finger between your own thumb

— and fingers (pincer movement).

Take a pause, one hand on the heart, the other on a wrist. Integrate.

THE FACE

There exists no real Tantric massage of the face. You may end

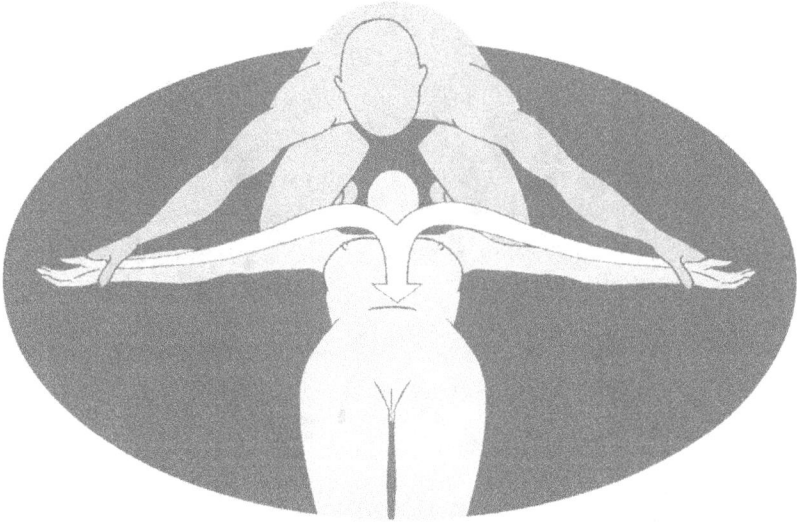

Figure 21. Arms and hands.

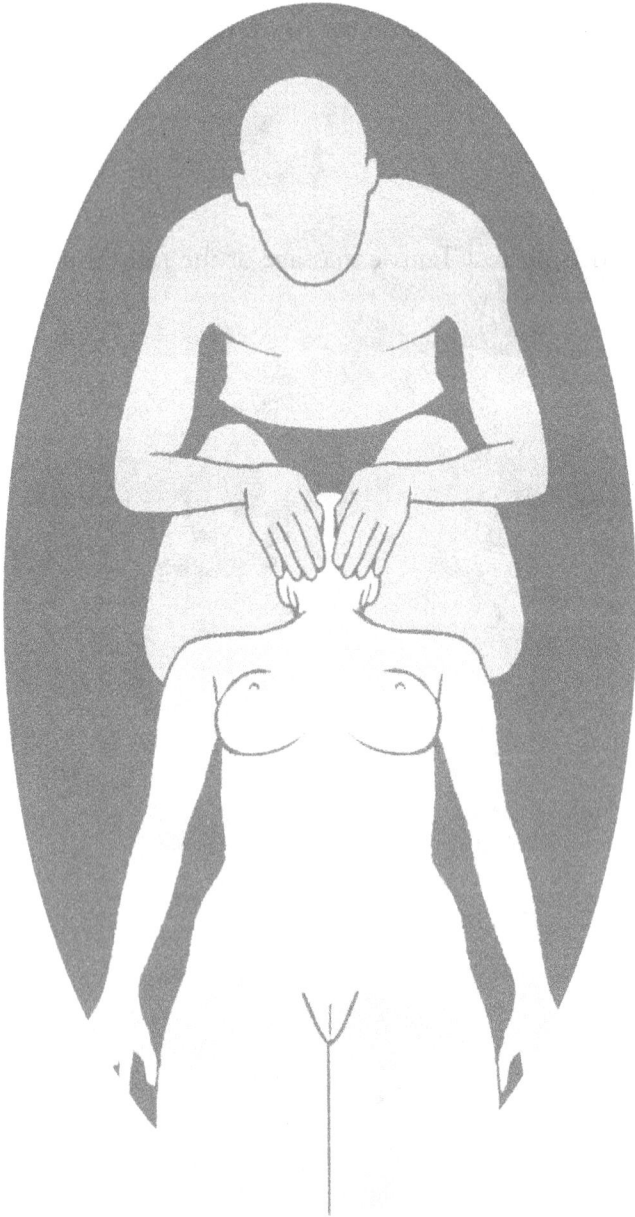

Figure 22. Ending the massage.

TANTRIC AND KASHMIRI MASSAGES

your massage now or supplement it with a facial massage as described in **Chapter 7** (Korean relaxation).

ENDING THE MASSAGE

Choose some movement in the previous chapter to close your massage. Leave the person to meditate in silence. You may remain kneeling behind their head or else you may sit there. The receiver will find you over them on opening their eyes.

My advice

When you have done two or three traditional massages in the axis of the kundalinî, you may glean some tips and new movements on the Tantric star-shaped massage in the previous chapter.

CHAPTER 13

KASHMIRI MASSAGE: GETTING READY

This form of massage draws its fundamentals directly from the Tantra as an agent of healing and connection. A person with no notion of massage can learn it quickly for the moves are simple and natural. On the other hand, achieving fluidity in the transitions between the different positions is not so easy and needs practice. The illustrations might help you to do this without breaking contact or disturbing the receiver's pleasant state.

The beginnings are often awkward. The persons you will be massing during a training session will forgive you since every beginner will experience the same difficulties. But so long as you are motivated and follow the instructions, you will perform a successful Kashmiri massage on the second or third try.

SEQUENCES

The two protocols are on offer, the complete sequence (five positions for the receiver) and the simple sequence (two positions), both have the advantage of suggesting a flow of movements which seems self-evident, especially when you have already practiced the Tantric massage. In both of these, the treatment of the ventral and dorsal areas is often synchronized with broad, simultaneous movements of both arms and hands. The massage of the different areas is punctuated with "freeze frames", a laying on of hands in one of the versions already discussed: the giver's hands placed on two distant chakras creating a current of energy which irrigates all the receiver's chakras. These pauses last from 10 to 15 seconds, then the giver "integrates" with long flowing strokes on the zone which has just been massaged during the globalization phase (see **Chapter 10**).

ACCESSORIES

A Kashmiri massage takes place on a mattress, futon or tatami placed on the floor and covered with towels and/or a sheet of oilcloth, like in the Tantric massage. We use a non-greasy scented massage oil. The amount of oil used varies considerably: some people spread it on like butter. Others prefer a more direct contact with the skin. (All the tips about the different styles of oiling are described in **Chapter 8**).

THE GIVER'S PREPARATION

The person giving the massage wears a pair of shorts or a bathing costume, and most of the time sits cross-legged or kneels. The pouring bottle is open and within easy reach at their side. Thus they can pour oil with one hand on the area to be massaged while the other hand keeps contact with the receiver's recumbent body. Hygiene and golden rules are the same as for a Tantric massage.

THE RECEIVER'S PREPARATION

Before the massage, the person will have taken a shower, which is a good way to clean the mind if one is coming from outdoors. According to arrangements made beforehand, the receiver will be naked or wearing some disposable undergarment, loose enough to allow one's partner to slip their hands beneath it. Their ventral breathing is like a baby's. It is also possible to breathe through the lower abdomen, as though one were trying to detach the muscles from the pubic bone. Thus the diaphragm grows more flexible and incites the rest of the body and mind to follow suit. This makes it easier for the receiver to cope with the emotions which may surface at any moment of the massage.

PRELIMINARY RITUAL

It is the same as for a Tantric massage and will last 10 minutes on the average (see **Chapter 10**).

Sitting crossed-legged face to face, join hands at heart-level and look into one another's eyes. Try to synchronize your breathing. You are now in close touch with your partner. After a few minutes, bow to each other, point your hands towards the floor. Keep the face to face posture in silence for a few minutes more in order to reach the peaceful concentration necessary for a massage. The giver can guide a receiver who is not familiar with the Tantra, providing instructions to loosen them up, or use the sound of a Tibetan bowl to raise the level of spirituality. (see Connecting with your partner in **Chapter 9**).

CHAPTER 14

THE COMPLETE SEQUENCE OF A KASHMIRI MASSAGE

Duration: 90 minutes

POSITION 1: YAB-YUM

This position will vary according to the degree of intimacy and confidence between the two partners. Some are close friends. Others form a couple, others are simply devoid of any taboos about intimate body contact, still others are already involved with this kind of massage or are already genuine Tantrikas. All of these may begin with the Yab-Yum, a tight embrace, pubis to pubis. If none of these situations apply, then you should begin with the following massage: the simple sequence (see **Chapter 15**).

You are sitting cross-legged or in the lotus position at one end of the futon or tatami, your oil-bottle to hand. The receiver comes and sits facing you between your thighs and wraps their legs around your hips but without crossing ankles: these must lie loosely behind the giver. Your two bodies are connected by the lower abdomen. This is the position known as Shakti and Shiva, as if you were going to engage in Tantric intercourse, but this is not the case! Whether you are giving or receiving the massage, do not let yourself be carried away by your fantasies! This contact is merely an exchange of energy. It is not a "carnal act". It can be perfectly well established between two straight people of the same sex. This connection will last throughout the massage with absolutely no sexual intention or excitation. Energy will begin to circulate between the energetic poles of the two of you if the massage is correctly executed, and there will be an input of energy on both sides. This connection may not be achieved the very first time, or it may be scrambled if the receiver is insufficiently relaxed, or if they are resistant to this kind of sharing.

— Begin with a rocking motion for as long as the Yab-Yum lasts: hold your partner in your arms for a few minutes with all the tenderness you feel for your own child. This reciprocal tenderness will open up the heart chakra.

OILING AND MASSAGING THE BACK

— Pour the oil into your palms and oil the back of the receiver sitting pressed against you, using both hands. At the same time, massage their back from bottom to top causing the energy to rise from the sacrum to the neck. Your hands should be enveloping, protective, loving. They slide one after the other. They may also rise and fall on both sides, symmetrically.

— Massage the back of the skull. Once the energy has reached the nape of the neck, bring it back down to the sacrum, the first chakra.

— Finish with a pause, one hand cupped over the sacrum and the other in the middle of the back, opposite the heart chakra or the solar plexus.

The pauses at each phase of the massage are meant to connect the receiver with the spiritual dimension and place them in a meditative state. The giver takes advantage of these pauses to straighten up and stretch their back.

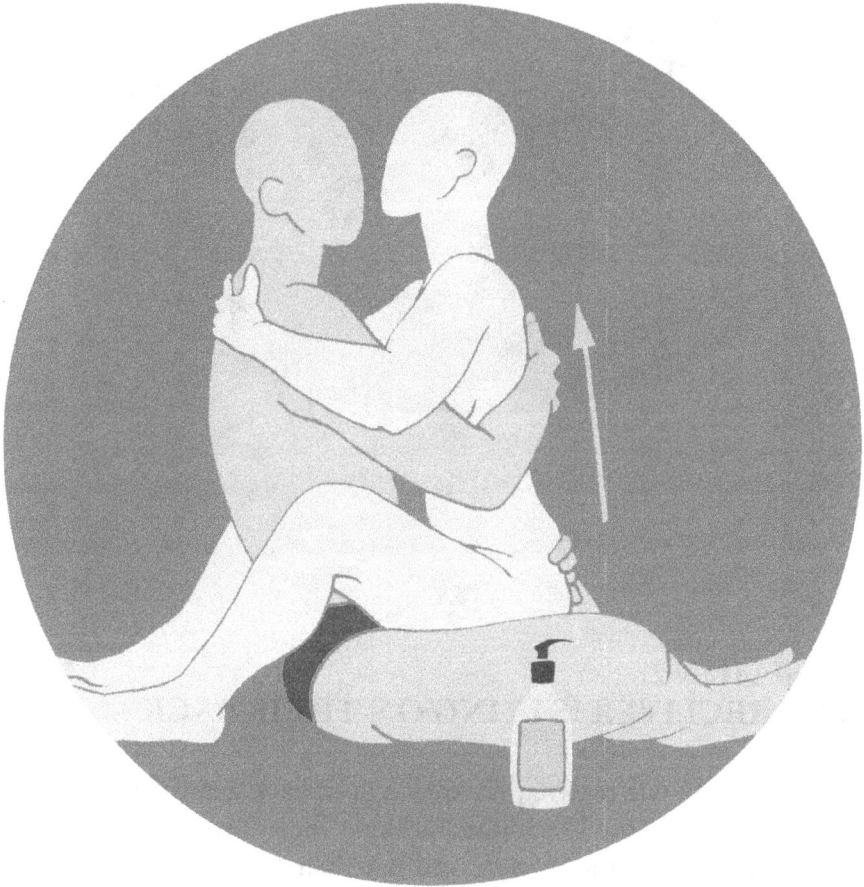

Figure 23. Yab-Yum.

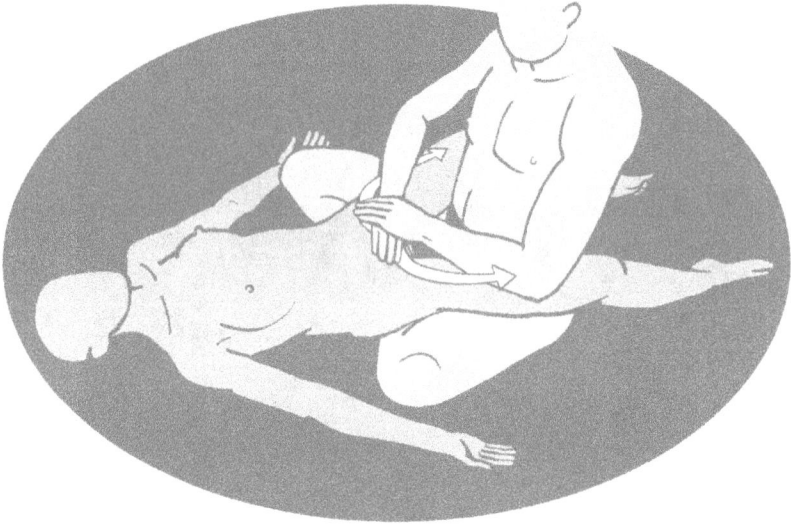

Figure 24. Pubis, thighs and legs.

POSITION 2:
THE RECEIVER IS LYING ON THEIR BACK

Supporting your receiver, lay their upper back gently on the oilcloth or bath-towels without breaking the contact between your two perinea: the receiver still has their legs behind your buttocks, relaxed and slightly bent, arms comfortably relaxed at their sides, or slightly spread, totally receptive. Their hipbone is still on your knees, or else it has slipped to the floor and their legs are further apart, as is more frequent. You may also move backwards: your receiver's legs will still be behind you but you will no longer have their buttocks on your knees and will no longer have to support their weight.

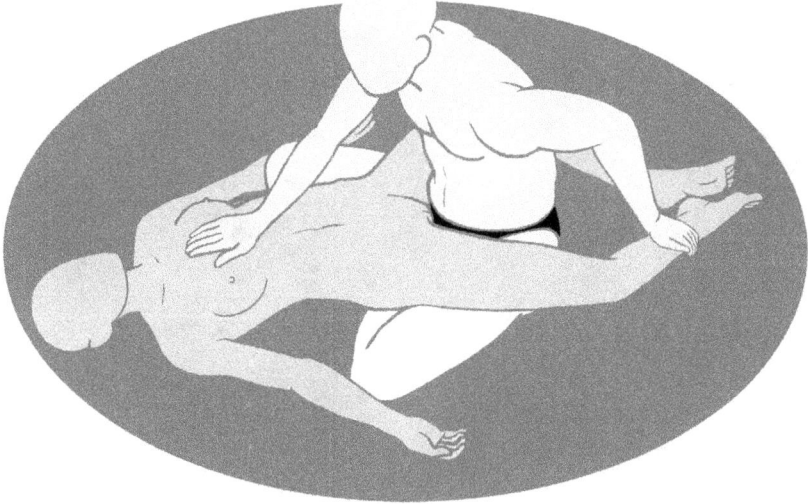

Figure 25. Laying on of hands.

MASSAGING THE PUBIS, THIGHS AND LEGS

➤ Pour a liberal amount of warm oil on the pubis and spread it to the groin, the lower abdomen and thighs. If you and your partner have already done this, massage from top to bottom and bottom to top, then the genitals briefly (see **Chapter 16**). Important: you must only punctuate your massage with brief, segmented massages of the genitals, they must not last for this might awaken the receiver's libido, as massaging the genitals is only meant to amplify the massage, create a bridge to the heart.

➤ If you are flexible enough, moisten the full length of the legs behind you with the oil. Both your hands should slide symmetrically over each limb if you can bend at the hips

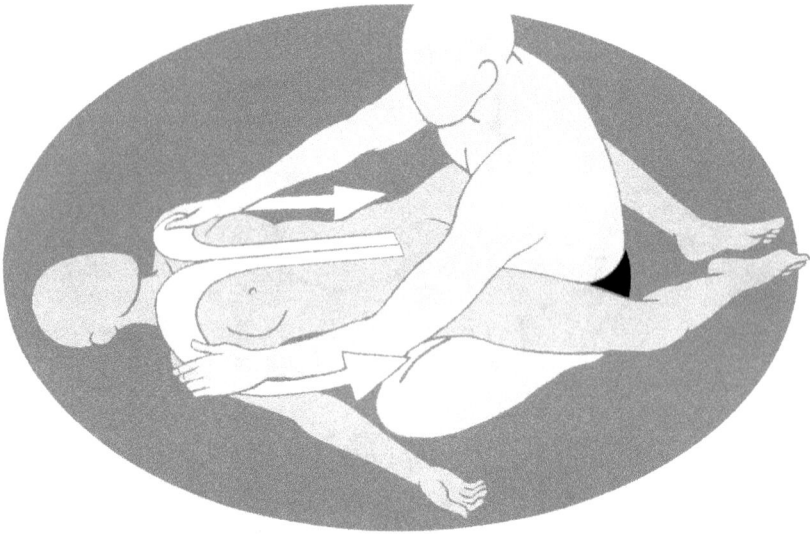

Figure 26. Torso and belly.

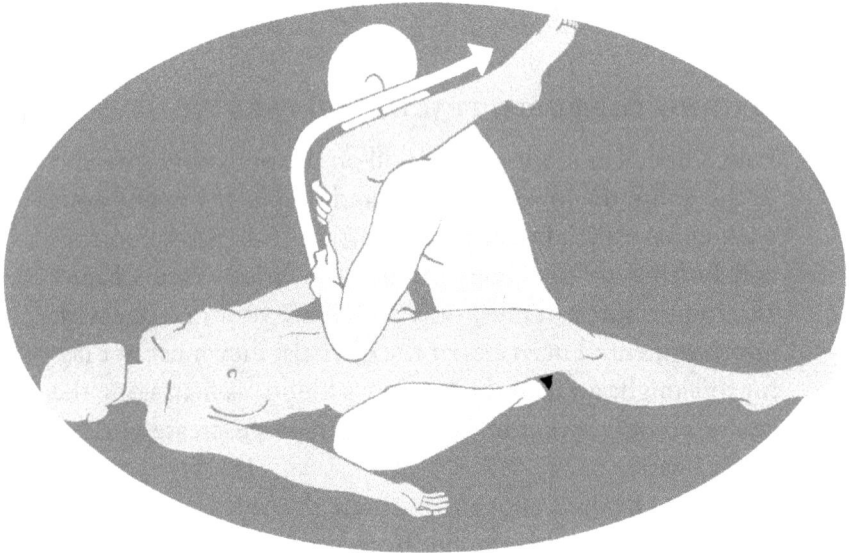

Figure 27. Legs.

TANTRIC AND KASHMIRI MASSAGES

sufficiently. If you can't manage it, massage the legs one at a time, swiveling slightly towards the leg in question, even if you have to lay the receiver's hips on the floor (if they are not already there) and back away.

➤ Take a pause, one hand on the heart, the other on an ankle.
➤ Integrate by spreading your hands.

TORSO AND ABDOMEN

With one hand, pour oil on the receiver's torso while keeping contact with the other. Spread the oil by massaging the belly in little circles without applying any pressure with your palm or fingers. If the receiver is a small person, you may lay one hand over the other. If your partner is a woman, be careful not to pull the skin on the lower abdomen upwards to avoid stimulating the genital area.

➤ Massage the heart and plexus chakras, then the throat chakra.
➤ Take a pause between each of these brief massages, keeping one hand on the chakra, the other on an ankle.
➤ Integrate by sliding both hands to the sternum, then up to the throat, before returning to the ankles by way of the abdomen in broad symmetrical sweeps. Such is the case each time we bring the energy upwards: we must then take it down again.
➤ Lift the receiver's body by the waist to deal with the rear ends of the ribs, massaging them upwards and downwards as well as the waist. You should give your partner the sensation that they are completely in your hands and perfectly weightless.

LEGS AND FEET

➤ Raise the receiver's leg up to your shoulder so as to have the sole of their foot within reach of your hand without having to writhe about uncomfortably. Massage the chakra in the center of the sole. Put the leg back down.
➤ Lift the other one onto your shoulder and massage it as well.

➤ Put it back on the oilcloth.
➤ Take a pause, one hand on the receiver's dantian, the other forms a clenched fist on the perineum.

Always massage at the same speed with no accelerations.

CHANGING THE RECEIVER'S POSITION

Turn your receiver over gently until they are lying flat on their stomach. This is not easy, all the less so if your partner is heavier than you. Ideally, you should be slightly to one side. Remove your partner's hips from your thighs if that is where they are placed. Slide over to their right side. Lift up their torso to place it first on their left side facing you, who are now sitting on their right side. Massage that near side with large, sweeping strokes before placing your partner face down.

POSITION 3:
THE RECEIVER IS LYING FACE DOWN

Take your partner's pelvis and lift it onto your thighs. To do this, slide one of your knees under the sacrum. Pull on their hips until your dantian is in contact with your partner's perineum. Your respective energies will thus communicate via this point throughout this stage of the massage. Lay your partner's arms alongside their body, spreading them slightly so they will be completely relaxed in that position. The receiver is now in the position known as the "Tantric wheelbarrow" which may prove uncomfortable for certain subjects. If you sense your partner is ill at ease, lower the hips from your thighs to the oilcloth. Take a pause, one hand on the heart chakra, the other on the sacrum.

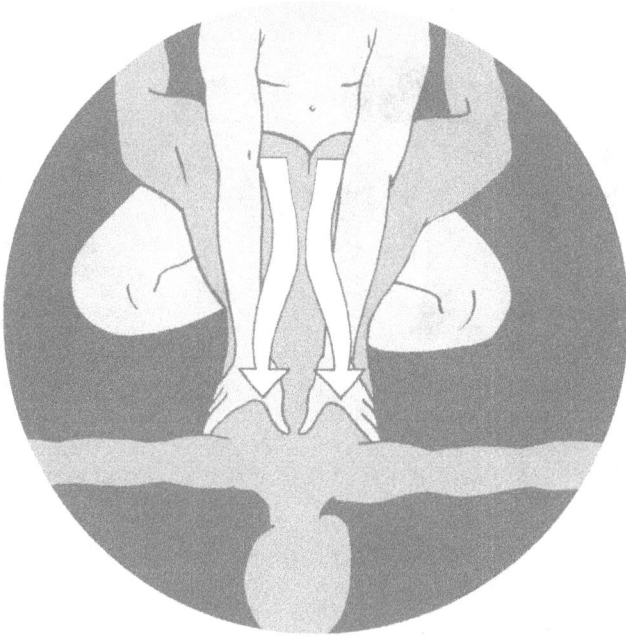

Figure 28. Back.

BACK, ARMS, BUTTOCKS AND LEGS

Oil the back if necessary, keeping contact with the other hand while picking up the bottle. This phase will enable you to integrate the previous sequence: you massage the whole body with broad strokes.

➤ The first sliding movements bring the energy up from the sacrum to the neck. You start from the buttocks and move towards the neck, massaging as well the back of the skull, three times.

➤ Massage the arms symmetrically up to the shoulders, then down to the wrists, three times as well.

➤ Massage the legs towards the rear with the fingers of both

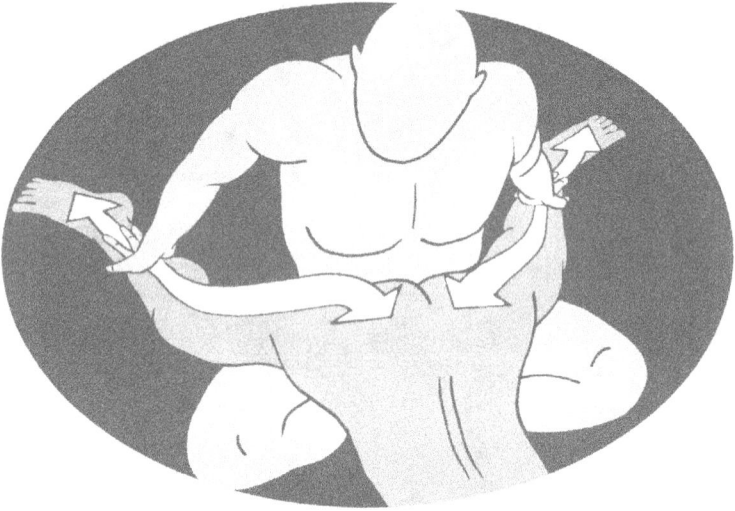

Figure 29. Buttocks and legs.

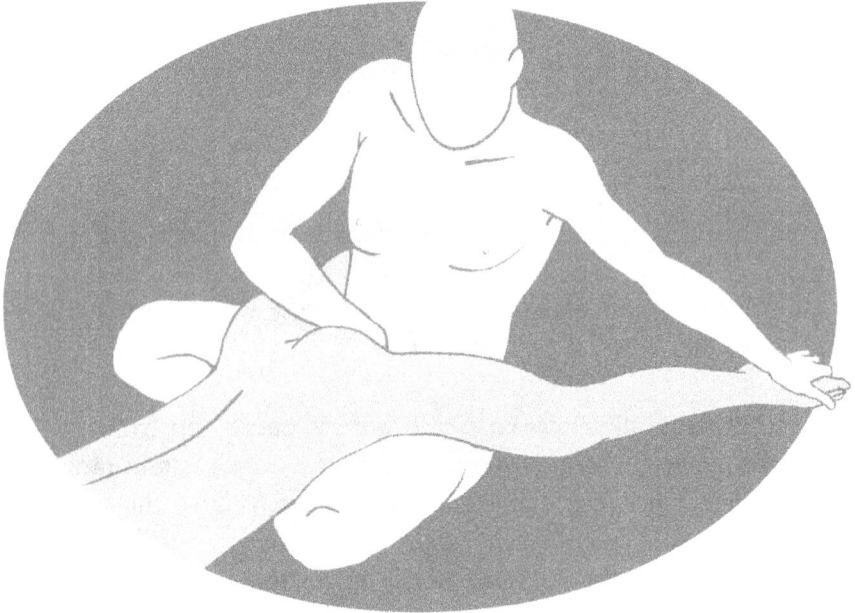

Figure 30. Laying on of hands (genitals, ankle).

　　　　　　　　　　　　TANTRIC AND KASHMIRI MASSAGES

hands pointing towards the feet and back again with the fingers pointing towards the buttocks in a smooth, symmetrical move.

➤ Bring the energy up and then down before taking a pause, with one hand on the receiver's ankle, the other on their genitals.

➤ If this is not your first massage nor your partner's, massage the genitals with your forearm slipped under her body if the receiver is a woman, pressed on the perinea if it is a man. If it has been agreed beforehand, you may undertake at this point a massage of a man's prostate or a woman's vulva, or her vagina (see **Chapter 16**).

➤ Finish with one hand on the genitals, the other on an ankle.

HOW TO CHANGE POSITIONS SUCCESSFULLY

With an eye to rolling your receiver onto their side (look at the **figures 15** and **16** in **Chapter 12**). Lift one of the arms and bend up the leg on the same side forming a right angle at the knee. This will give easy access to the receiver's genitals and will facilitate a brief massage of these, always provided it has been agreed beforehand that they are to be included. Roll the receiver onto their side holding the hips and torso. One of your thighs will be in contact with the person's buttocks, the other with the underside of their thighs.

THE RECEIVER IS NOW IN POSITION 4:

LYING ON THEIR RIGHT SIDE IN A FOETAL POSITION

Which positions favor genital massage ?

In the traditional Tantric massage, when the receiver is on their back you are between their thighs, on your knees or sitting cross-legged. In a Kashmiri massage you are sitting cross-legged against their buttocks. It is at this stage of the massage that you can deal with the genitals as in **Chapter 16**. This is also possible when the person is lying face down and you lift their pelvis onto your thighs, reversing the position of the Tantric wheelbarrow.

HIPS, ARMS, THIGHS

— Leave your hands cupped for a few moments on the receiver's hips in order to calm their energy after this transition.
— Oil their side while your other hand keeps the contact. Spread the oil with broad movements including the left arm, top and bottom, but also the inside of the right arm on the floor.
— Keep your fingers together exerting an even pressure with the whole hand. Firmly wrap both hands around their thighs and knees.
— Integrate with one hand on the sacrum, the other on the dantian.

SIMULTANEOUS MASSAGE OF THE BACK AND TORSO

The advantage of the foetal position is to be able to reach the front and back of the torso at the same time.

- Bring the energy up from the sacrum to the neck as you did from the starting position. Your hands must move with perfect symmetry on both sides. If you need to add oil on the front of the torso, make sure you maintain contact with the other hand.
- Finish with a pause, one hand on the sacrum, the other on the heart chakra, between the pectoral muscles.
- Reverse the positions of your hands for a integration with broad, sweeping strokes, the hand that was massaging the back now massages the chest and vice versa.
- Then reverse the positions of the hands and take a pause.

LEGS

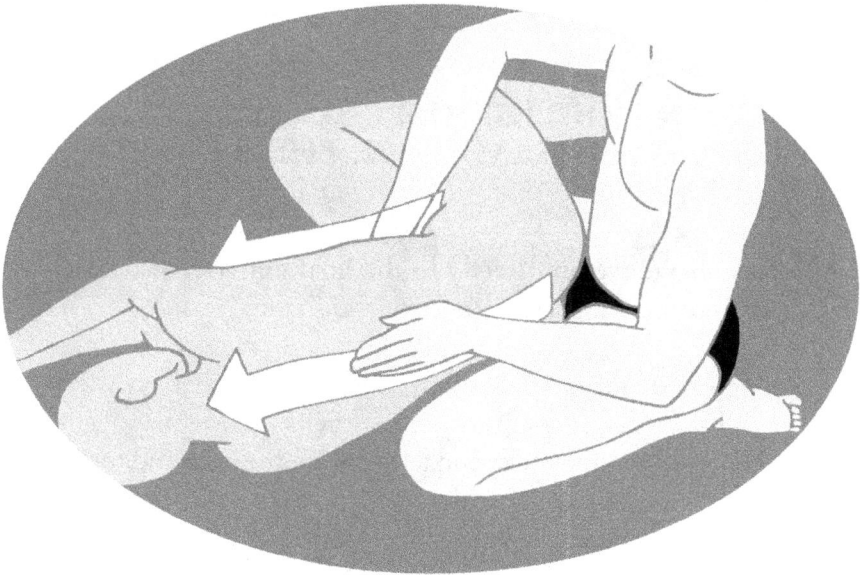

Figure 31. Back and torso.

- Massage with short strokes the leg on the uppermost side. One hand follows the other all the way to the receiver's ankle.
- Take another pause, one hand on the heart, the other on the sacrum.
- Integrate the massage with broad strokes over the whole leg.

If you wish, you may finish with another pause, one hand on the ankle, the other on the thigh or hip.

Now bend the receiver's leg and place their foot flat on the floor.

- Massage the inside of the leg from the ankle to the crotch, one hand following the other.
- Take a pause. Integrate with broad strokes before finishing this phase with another pause, one hand on the ankle, the other on the heart chakra.

Gently straighten the leg and lay it back on the floor.

POSITION 5 (OPTIONAL): THE RECEIVER IS LYING ON THEIR LEFT SIDE

You may also move on directly to the final position of relaxation, thereby limiting the number of transitions.

Placing one hand on their right hip and the other on their torso, roll the receiver over onto their other side. The massage is the same as before, but you spend less time on the back and torso. Finish this stage with your hands cupped one on top of the other, over the heart chakra.

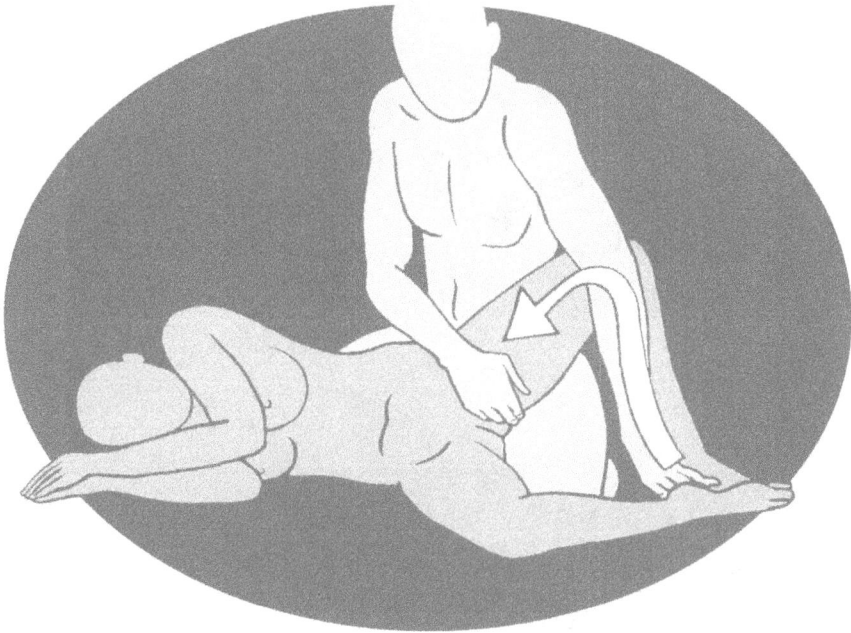

Figure 32. Legs.

FINISHING THE MASSAGE

Lay your partner on their back. Use the yin touch to finish the massage, with a silky cloth for example, or brushing the skin with your fingertips. There are several ways to close the massage. (**See** Massaging the face in **chapter 7**, or Ending the massage in **Chapter 11**). Cover the receiver with a towel. Allow a quarter of an hour for the infusion.

CHAPTER 15

THE SIMPLER SEQUENCE OF A KASHMIRI MASSAGE

Duration: 90 minutes

This sequence involves only two positions. Thus you limit the number of transitions for which a certain familiarity and a good flexibility are preferable. It also allows you to avoid an overly intimate contact with a person you do not know very well or not at all if this is a training session or a professional massage. Professional masseuses will often adopt this simpler succession with strangers rather than beginning with the Yab-Yum They will start by relaxing the receiver by massaging their side instead.

This very simple protocol allows beginners to work on the enveloping massage and develop the love they are going to try to transmit with their hands. Integration, with broad sliding strokes, will enable you to spread their sexual energy to the receiver's whole body.

POSITION 1:
LYING ON THE RIGHT SIDE

Place your receiver on the right side as not so compress their heart (located on the left side), curled up on the cloth or the towels. The slightly bent position of their legs will make it easy for your hands to reach every area. Sit on your heels next to their hips or buttocks. If necessary, you can shift your position in case you are not flexible enough at the waist to reach all the areas. Some independent masseuses use a low prayer stool during this first stage to spare their knees.

You may very well confine yourself to massaging one of your partner's sides since the face down position which follows will allow you to reach the areas you have missed, such as, for instance, the right arm and right side, which are pressed to the floor during this first phase.

THE RECEIVER IS LYING THREE-QUARTERS ON THEIR CHEST

OILING AND MASSAGING THE BACK, SHOULDERS AND BUTTOCKS

Use a generous amount of oil on the receiver's back.

- Move both hands together from the sacrum to the neck to bring the energy up. Massage the back of the skull as well. If you sense tension in your subject, knead their neck and trapezoid muscles in order to facilitate the rest of the massage, but don't make too much of this.
- Move on to the shoulders with both hands synchronized. Put all the love you can into the broad, enveloping movements of your hands. They may either slide one after the other, or move in opposite directions and join together again towards the small of the back. Both fingers and palms apply the same firm pressure.

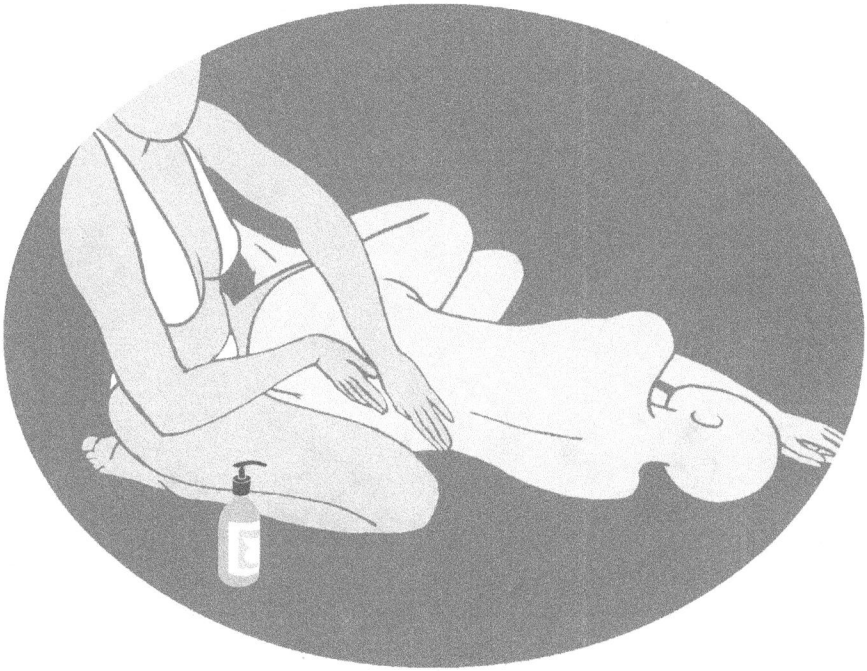

Figure 33. Back, shoulders, and buttocks

> Back away to massage the lower part. Then bring the energy down to the sacrum, the first chakra, the cradle of the kundalinî. Massage the buttocks firmly.
> Finish with a laying on of hands on the sacrum.

MASSAGING THE BELLY

Move the receiver's uppermost leg slightly off the other so as to reach the belly, the torso and both legs easily.

> Add oil on your hands to massage the belly in small circles, still with enveloping movements.
> Run your hands over the pubis, crotch and genitals but without lingering there: you do not avoid the genitals in

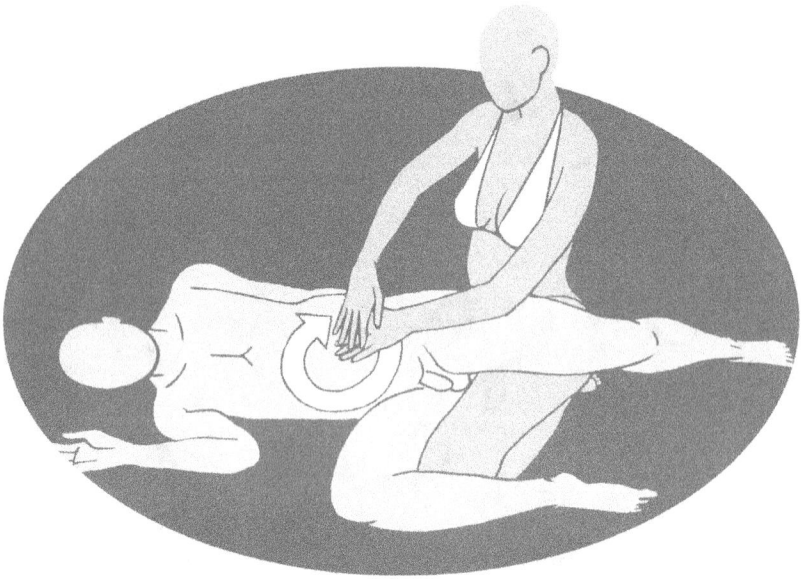

Figure 34. Belly.

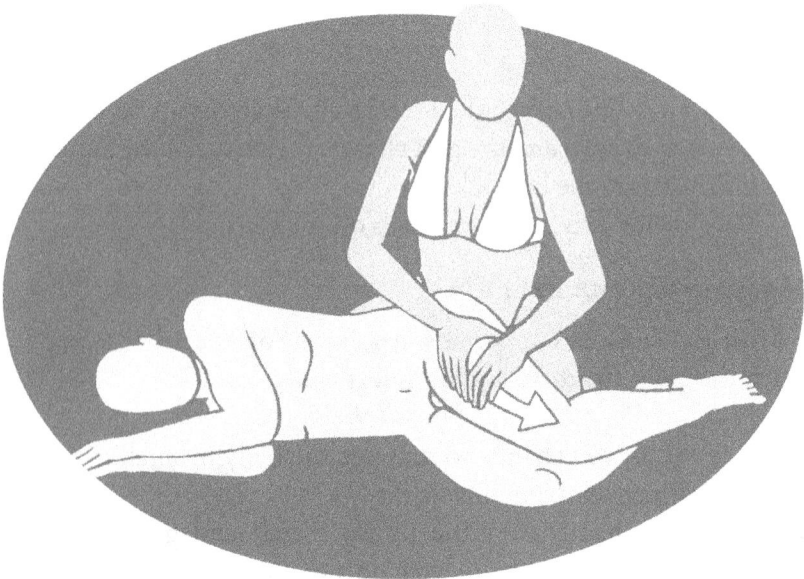

Figure 35. Thigh and leg.

TANTRIC AND KASHMIRI MASSAGES

these overall massages the way you do for an Ayurvedic massage, another type of massage for which oil can be used in abundance.

— Take a pause, one hand on the middle of the back opposite the heart, the other on the pubis or genitals.

MASSAGING THE TORSO

— Run your hands between the pectoral muscles or breasts, over the sternum and then down both sides, symmetrically.
— Finish with a laying on of hands, one on the pubis, the other on the heart.

MASSAGING THE THIGHS AND THE LEGS

Spread oil on the thighs and legs.

— Massage the whole length of the legs towards the feet, you may need to move down alongside the receiver.

It doesn't matter if your torso touches the receiver while bending over: this benevolent intimacy is an integral part of a Tantric or Kashmiri massage. Between two people who know each other or who form a couple, your massage may be more intimate by pressing against your partner without it's becoming sexy for all that: tenderness is part of the massage.

MASSAGING THE FEET

— Massage the feet, from the edge to the middle, then the hollow behind the pad back of the big toe.
— Integrate by massaging with broad strokes the receiver's uppermost leg and side, and then their other leg and side.
— Take another pause, holding an ankle in one hand with the other resting on your receiver's sacrum (see The complete massage of the feet in **Chapter 7**).

POSITION 2:
LYING FACE DOWN

This transition is not an easy matter, all the more so as the receiver is now so relaxed from the previous stage that they risk emerging from their present state. Here is how to go about it. Sit cross-legged. Roll them over on their pelvic region. Slide closer to them and pull their legs towards you so as to press your lower abdomen against theirs with their pelvis resting on your knees. This is the Tantric wheelbarrow. You are now in contact with your partner's root chakra which is pressed against your lower abdomen. Pull their arms apart so that they will be more receptive to your massage.

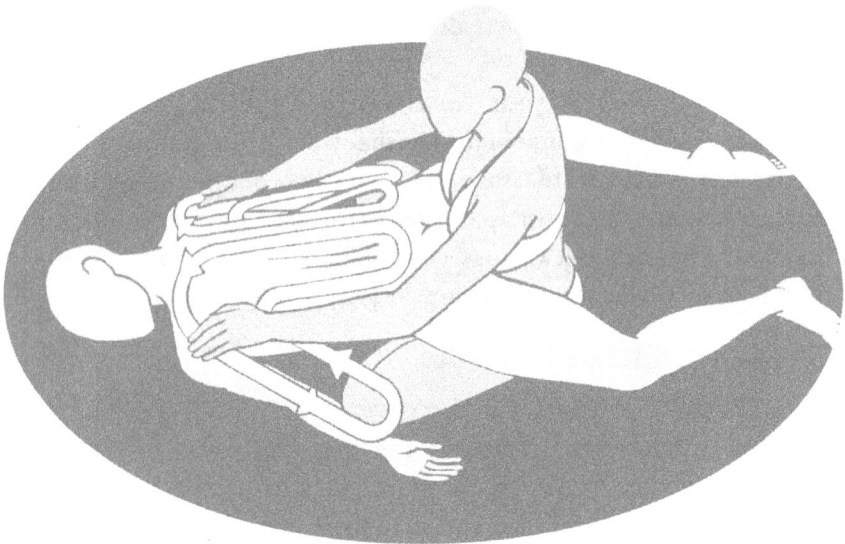

Figure 36. Back and arms.

TANTRIC AND KASHMIRI MASSAGES

MASSAGING THE BACK AND ARMS

➤ Spread oil on the back if necessary, slide both hands, one behind the other, up and down the spine at least three times, then use abdomen.

➤ Pull their arms apart so that they will be more receptive to your massage. further sliding movements with your hands and arms on the receiver's skin in order to bring the energy up from the sacrum to the nape of the neck as you did at the beginning of the massage.

➤ Massage one arm down to the fingers and take a pause with both hands cupped over these. Then massage the other arm.

➤ Take a pause keeping one hand on their wrist or the back of their hand, the other on their sacrum.

MASSAGING THE GENITALS (OPTIONAL)

➤ Next, massage the hips with symmetrical, enveloping movements. If permitted by your degree of intimacy, or by a previous agreement between your partner and yourself, massage their anus and possibly their genitals by passing your forearm under their raised pelvis (see **Chapter 16**). This stage must not be included in a first massage or a training session.

➤ Withdraw gently and lay your receiver's pelvis delicately on the floor. Continue the massage with sliding movements.

➤ With one hand, lift one of their knees, then the corresponding arm. This will make it easy to spread their thighs and turn the receiver on their back to let the massage sink in.

ENDING THE MASSAGE

You may use either the yin touch, brushing your hand over the skin (see **Chapter 11**) or a facial massage (see **Chapter 7**). Cover the receiver with a warm towel. Let the massage sink in for a quarter of an hour or so.

CHAPTER 16

MASSAGE
OF THE GENITALS

The genitals are massaged in order to confer upon these body parts, which we generally neglect except for the giving and taking of sexual pleasure, the presence, the contact and the attention they deserve. This massage may be part of a total massage or carried out on its own at some special moment, by a Tantrika of either sex or a person aspiring to achieve Tantric sexuality. The receiver of the massage is not meant to be aroused or to be holding back a sexual discharge of the ejaculatory type. A massage of our yoni (vulva) or lingam (penis) helps to balance our internal forces. Addressed thus at the level of our sex and sacrum, our sexual energy will spread to our organs and our chakras, providing them with nourishment. A feeling of plenitude gradually comes over the receiver. In this type of massage, an immediate comprehension of oneself is attained bodily rather than mentally. It is therefore essential to let go. Knowing our genitals as well as we know the rest of our body provides an anchorage, an equilibrium, a quiet, joyful strength.

A massage of the genitals never takes place during a first Tantric massage. It is far better to have tried your hand at several massages before including the genitals, and this applies to the receiver as well as to the giver. They must have a conversation beforehand to decide whether or not to include the genitals. Between partners who do not know one another —and even within a couple— any confusion with an erotic massage will make the receiver neglect the energy work characteristic of the Tantra, but also the meditative side. A good understanding of the Tantra is preferable in order to maintain the emotional and energetic aspects of the massage. Thus we can avoid any arousal which is likely to focus the receiver's attention on their genitals and sexual desire.

You may massage the genitals briefly at various moments during the massage. It's up to you to improvise when a favorable position occurs. For example in the case of a male receiver, when he is lying on his back, but also during the retroversion of the pelvis when he is on his stomach, or when his abdomen is resting on your thighs in the wheelbarrow position.

A genital massage is slow and meditative. It allows the receiver to identify their organs one by one and to re-appropriate them. It improves sexual performance and makes it possible to direct one's sexual energy inwards and draw nourishment from it.

You may divide your genital massage between the following stages, according to your partner's position.

WHEN THE RECEIVER IS LYING ON THEIR BACK

After the leg massage, slide between your partner's thighs. Or you may want to sit cross-legged to one side as in the Tantric massage for beginners and lay the receiver's nearest leg on your thigh.

A variant:

Slide over the cloth and lift the receiver's pelvis so as to rest their sacrum on your knees. Your pubis or your dantian is facing or pressed against their perineum.

When the receiver is lying face down

You are sitting cross-legged between your partner's thighs. Lift their pelvis onto your thighs in the wheelbarrow position. Massaging the genitals is done from below, with your hand and forearm.

IF THE RECEIVER IS A WOMAN

When she is lying on her back, one splayed leg resting on your thigh.

Thighs, crotch, pubis and vulva

- Oil the pubis. Begin with a pause, one hand on the belly, the other resting motionless on the sex. This is the moment of reassuring recognition, of one's total presence to the receiver when she becomes aware of her genitals. Synchronize your breathing with your partner's, deep breaths with your mouth open.
- Describe slow circles on the lower abdomen and then the crotch, with your hands in opposition or moving symmetrically.
- Massage the thighs while keeping your other hand on the pubis, then massage the pubis with upward strokes, then downward ones.
- Take a pause, with your hands at the top of the inside of each thigh, close to the groin, on those "iron doors" as Chinese doctors call these parts of the body which can sometimes block the libido. (See **Karsai nei tsang massage, Chapter 18**).
  Slide the pads of your fingers over the outside of the closed labia majora keeping the other hand on the pubis. Repeat this three times.
- Massage the outside of the vulva with the pads of your fingers keeping the labia majora shut.

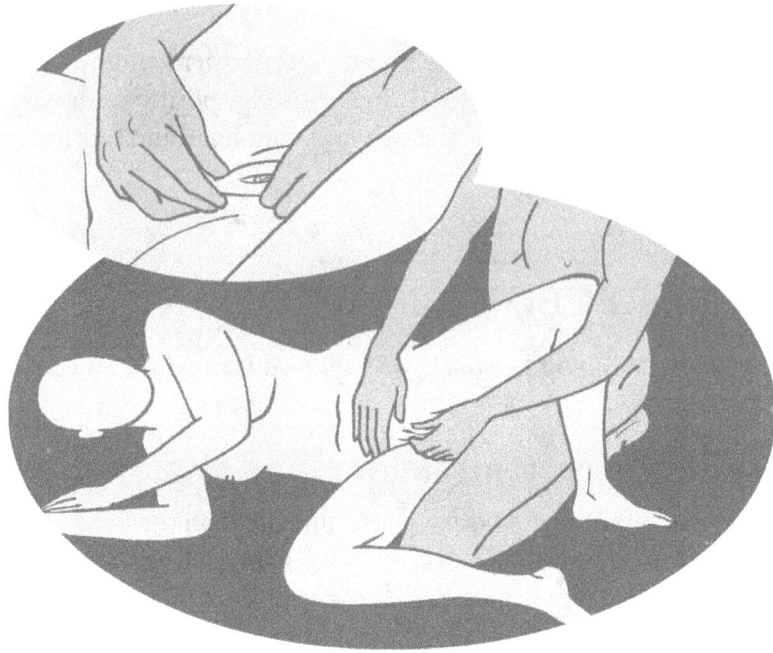

Figure 37-38. Massaging the genitals.

— Now practice the same slow, delicate move on the inner face of the majora. Repeat this.
— Keeping one hand on the pubis, spread the labia minora upwards while sliding your fingers slowly over them.
— Repeat the above with a different pressure.
— Take a pause, pressing two fingers on the high end of the vulva, where the labia minora separate at the base of the pubis. Meanwhile, your other hand is describing slow circles on the belly and the pubis.
— Now comes a laying on of hands, one on the closed vulva, the other on the receiver's ankle.

Vagina, anus and buttocks

- You may also insert two fingers into the vagina and leave them there without moving while you trace circles on the pubis. The goal here is to take the sexual energy into the abdomen and give it greater depth, rather than leaving it on and around the clitoris. Leave your fingers (or knuckles) where they are while you close the labia majora with the other hand.
- Withdraw your fingers and move down to the anus. Exert prolonged pressure on the perineum, just before the anal orifice. Relax the rim of the anus by massaging the inner faces of the buttocks with the palms of you hands, symmetrically, then again press on the perineum.
- Slide both hands up to the sternum, one hand following the other to diffuse the energy.
- Finish with one hand cupped over the genitals, the other on the heart. Put the receiver 's leg back in place.

In this position, you may choose to massage the woman's breasts.

When she is lying on her side, legs together

The massage can be done from behind and will involve the same moves for the vulva, even though the labia minora are less easily accessible from there. One may finish the massage with a laying on of hands, one on the perineum, the other on an ankle.

When she is lying face down, her pelvis on your thighs in the position of the Tantric wheelbarrow

- Massage the crotch, the cleft between the buttocks, and the perineum with broad firm strokes.
- Run one finger around the rim of the anus, briefly press the orifice two or three times.

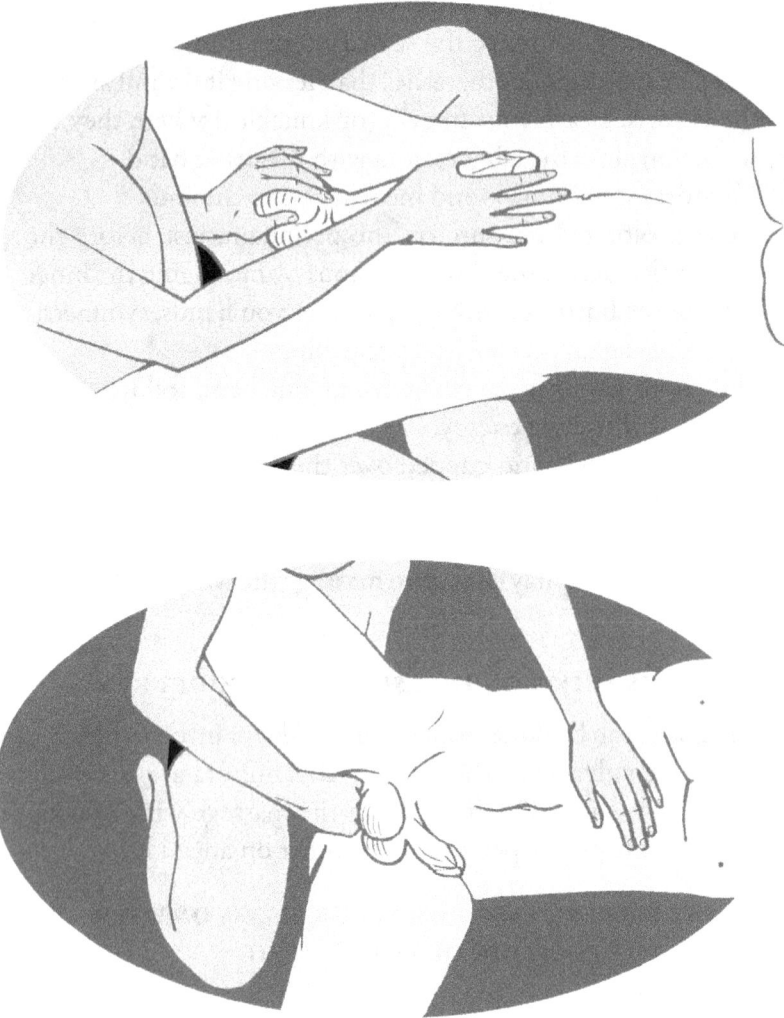

Figure 39-40. Massaging the genitals.

- Slip your forearm beneath her belly. Brush the back of your hand or your palm over the labia majora while continuing to press with your hands or your knuckles the edge of the vulva.
- Repeat the brushing movement.
- Slowly withdraw both hands.
- Integrate by massaging her waist symmetrically with broad enveloping movements and passing your arms under her belly from the sides.
- Take a pause, one hand over the heart, the other on the perineum.

Read if necessary the passages dealing with the perineum and the anatomy of female and male genitals (see Chapter 20).

IF THE RECEIVER IS A MAN

WHEN HE IS LYING ON HIS BACK, HIS PELVIS RESTING ON THE PELVIS OF THE WOMAN SITTING CROSS-LEGGED

- Moisten his pubis with oil. Cup one hand over his genitals, the other on his belly, and take a pause. Synchronize your breathing, with your mouth open.
- Massage his belly with gentle rotations, one hand following the other.
- Now your hand slides under his testicles and penis, the top of the thighs and the crotch slowly and without exerting pressure (yin touch). Run one hand over the perineum and the anus, without lingering.
- Take a pause, one hand on the solar plexus, the other on the perineum.
- Integrate by massaging down one leg and up the other.
- Take the penis in both hands and hold it to ensure a first contact. One hand at the level of the glans (but with no traction on the foreskin which must remain closed while the

other hand slowly massages the shaft up and down. Extend your manipulations around the testicles and slowly massage the crotch. By enveloping the testicles, you bring the energy downwards.

- Take a pause, one hand on the hamp, the other on the perineum.
- Integrate by massaging the belly and the inner face of the thighs.
- Finish with one hand over the heart, the other on the hamp.
- Delicately bring together the receiver's legs.

WHEN HE IS LYING ON HIS SIDE AS IN A KASHMIRI MASSAGE

You are kneeling to the rear of his buttocks and you twist his torso just enough so that his back is flat on the cloth. Lifting his upper leg will make it easier to reach his genitals. Lay his foot flat on the cloth. The massage of the genitals is the same as above.

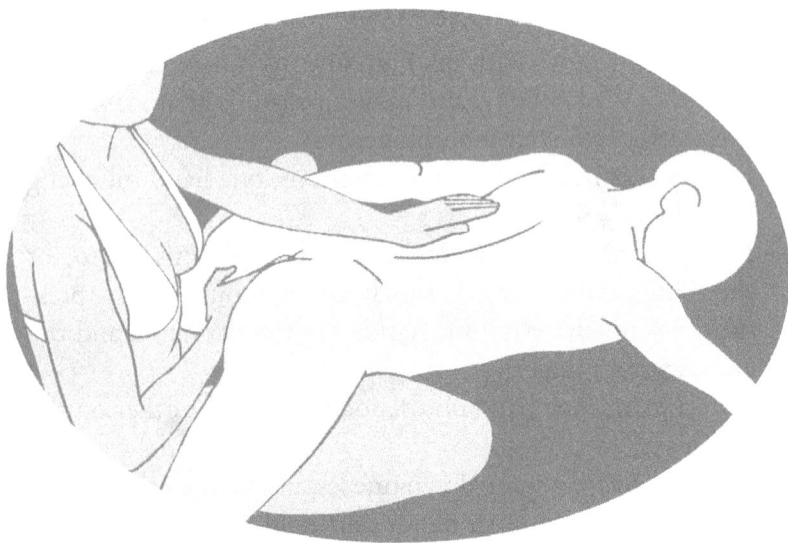

Figure 41. Massaging the anus, for a woman or a man.

WHEN HE IS LYING FACE DOWN, WITH HIS PELVIS ON YOUR THIGHS IN THE WHEELBARROW POSITION

Warm the sacrum with both hands for a few seconds. Pour a little oil high on the buttocks. Massage the perineum, then the testicles with your thumbs from below, symmetrically, move around them, cradle them in your hands. Repeat each move two or three times.

- With one hand on his penis, bring the energy up to the nape of his neck with the other hand. Massage the penis with a firm hand (yang touch) making no effort to excite him. Hold it with both hands long enough for a firm kneading-rolling.
- Run your thumbs along both sides of the anal zone in order to distend the rim. Press both sides symmetrically with your palms or your knuckles.
- Leave the edge of your hand, motionless, between the buttocks, sunk between the anus and the perineum, while with the other hand you bring the energy up along the spine to the neck.
- Slip your arms beneath both of his sides and massage the penis with both hands.
- Withdraw your hands and bring the energy up on both sides of the spine and then bring it down again.
- Integrate with broad strokes on the small of the back and the legs.
- Take a pause with three fingers on the perineum and the other hand on the scrotum.

If the receiver has an erection, spread his energy with broad, slow strokes on the legs and thighs and move on to the next stage.

MASSAGING YOUR OWN GENITALS

Duration: 20 to 40 minutes

Requisites

- Atmospheric lighting
- A bath-towel
- Essential oils in a diffuser

This involves taking some time alone to take care of yourself, for our genitals are part of our most precious possession, our body, our conveyance. Keeping our genitals on the qui vive is a guarantee of good health, energy and pleasure. But mind you: this is not masturbation. Avoid sex-toys and quick, jerky movements. And take your time!

- Lying on comfortable cushions, legs slightly apart, apply a bit of oil to your pubis. Moisten the inner face of your thighs symmetrically with both hands.
- Run the pads of your fingers along each side of your organ, slowly, then over the genitals without lingering.
- Massage your belly in small circles, then your hips, the sides and bottoms of your thighs.
- Cup your hand over your genitals, breathe slowly and deeply, imagining you are breathing through them. Breathe out through your mouth. Repeat three times.
- Now with both hands return to your crotch. Spread your thighs in a V, massage their inner faces at length, those areas which the Chinese call the "iron doors" because they can paralyze the libido if a person has blockages (often psychological) in the lower abdomen. You will begin to feel excited, which is perfectly normal.
- Move away from the genital area. Massage your breasts in circles with the pads of your fingers.

— Now spread your thighs further and move your hands to your anus. This is the area where anger and frustration accumulate. Massage the rim of the anus, the inner faces of the buttocks on each side with the whole palm until you feel this area starting to relax. With broad strokes, diffuse into your belly all the energy which you have just liberated.

IF YOU ARE A WOMAN

— Massage the labia majora, the outside and the inside, slowly and firmly.

IF YOU ARE A MAN

— massage the penis and testicles with broad, firm and enveloping movements. Do this again slowly.
— If you feel energy concentrated in the genitals (tip of the glans or clitoris, testicles, vaginal entrance, labia minora, etc.) disseminate it by massaging a larger region, the inner faces of your thighs, your belly and torso, and with your breathwork induce it to circulate.

Leave one hand cupped over your genitals and slide the other to your heart. Close your eyes and let it infuse.

My advice to women

Avoid massaging your clitoris. A Tantric genital massage is never intended to produce a clitoral orgasm, often a source of irritation afterwards, or tension in the lower abdomen. True pleasure lies deep in the vagina, the rectum and the vestigial prostate behind the G-spot, in other words in the innermost depths of your body, and will provide you with far more energy than a superficial orgasm.

CHAPTER 17

THERAPEUTIC MASSAGE

Duration: 40 minutes

This massage is meant to awaken our roots, the cradle of the Kundalinî and the base of the spine, the first chakra. It is unnecessary to use a great deal of oil. One can even massage the back without any oil at all. But it is best to use some when massaging the perineum.

If you are about to receive a massage, the time is ripe for you to admit... that your orgasms are very rare/that it takes an infinite amount of time to have one/that you have never had an orgasm/ or on the contrary (if you are a man) that you ejaculate as soon as your penis is touched.

If you are giving the massage, this is the time to ask questions like: "are there parts of your body which are painful and which I must massage more gently? Are there positions that are uncomfortable for you?"

If the person that you are about to massage suffers from a blockage, temporary impotence or inhibitions, don't hesitate to ask them when they had their last orgasm. Such questions make for a certain intimacy, of the kind encountered in a doctor's office, an intimacy peculiar to this one situation and which ends when you take leave of one another in the case of a professional massage.

THE RECEIVER IS LYING FACE DOWN, THE GIVER IS KNEELING BESIDE THEM

Your naked partner lies face down on a futon covered with a large beach towel, their forehead on their hands, breathing deeply. You, wearing underclothes, are on your knees beside the receiver.

➤ Execute broad strokes on their back with your forearms, applying only moderate, equal pressure with the fingers and palms. Loosen up the neck and the shoulders with broad strokes, then move down the spine to release the tension on both sides of each vertebrae, massaging in tight circles the points that seem tense.

Exert light pressure each time your partner exhales, exhaling at the same time yourself. You should hear them breathe out when you exert light pressure on their back. Release your pressure each time their exhalation ends but leaving your hand in contact with the skin. Synchronizing your breathing will establish communication between you.

THE GIVER BETWEEN THE RECEIVER'S LEGS

Settle between your partner's legs, sitting on your heels or on the floor.

➤ Exert pressure below the waist where the adrenal glands are located in order to stimulate their secretions and the receiver's sexual responses.
➤ Massage the legs symmetrically to the feet with broad sliding strokes, first downwards and then upwards, finally bringing the energy to the sacrum.

Pull the receiver's sacrum onto your thighs in the wheelbarrow position.

IF YOU ARE MASSAGING A WOMAN

➤ Use both hands to describe a triangle starting from the middle of the back opening out around the buttocks. Massage her several times according to this pattern, keeping your hands flat.

➤ Grasp her hips with both hands and gently rotate them several times. Slide your hands under her pelvis and massage the pubis.

➤ According to what has been agreed beforehand, you may massage her genitals as in **Chapter 16**, including the labia majora and minora.

IF YOU ARE DEALING WITH A MAN

➤ Massage the perineum and testicles.

Then you may rest for a while, leaning on your partner's shoulder in a surge of affection, if you have a close relationship.

THE RECEIVER IS LYING ON THEIR BACK

Next, ask your partners to turn over and lie on their back, helping them if necessary. Lift their pelvis onto your thigh, in the same position they were in when lying face down.

➤ Again gently rotate their pelvis, synchronizing your breathing with theirs. A sexual blockage is often located here. Massage in circles around the navel and the pelvis.

All of these movements are light and gentle but must not be mistaken for erotic caresses. (See The art of touch in **Chapter 6**). Their vibrant action is intended to awaken the erogenous zones in the nether regions of the body. The love you put into your hands is an essential component of the Kashmiri massage.

If the receiver is a man

➣ You may follow up with a massage of the prostate, provided you have agreed on this beforehand. (See Prostate massage in Chapter 20). Otherwise, massage slowly and gently the perineal area and the rim of the anus.

If you are dealing with a woman

➣ Massage slowly the labia of the vulva, keeping them closed, once from top to bottom, then two or three times up to her crotch.

Finish with a pause, one hand cupped over the receiver's genitals (his lingam or her yoni) the other on the dantian.

CHAPTER 18

ENERGY MASSAGE OF THE BELLY, THE LOWER ABDOMEN AND GENITALS: KARSEI NEI TSANG

Duration: 30 minutes

This massage differs from the previous one in that it acts upon the workings of our bodily fluids and meridians, like many techniques originating in China. This is an ancient Taoist massage meant to stimulate the circulation in the lower parts of the body, the blood returning to the heart through the veins. The karsai nei tsang opens our vessels, softens the walls of our veins, improves the flow of energy in our belly and lower abdomen and helps evacuate various residua (toxins, sediments). It cleanses the "second brain" by eliminating the waste that causes worries and fears (lodged in the spleen), phobias and traumas (lodged in the kidneys), jealousy, frustrations and anger (lodged in the liver).

Thus it enables a person to anchor their body and their energy in the pelvic region, their deepest support, the first chakra. Indeed, the second part of the karsai, the massage of the perineum and the genitals, is meant for people who have difficulty feeling their perineum, or who are not anchored in depth. A Tantric procedure will enable them to retain the openness acquired through the karsai and to reappropriate their genitals at the psychological and affective levels. People over fifty who have difficulties becoming aroused, or others in whom arousal weakens during intercourse will find their genital energy increased thanks to the improvement of their circulation.

FIRST STEPS

The videos of the Sino-Thai doctor Mantak Chia, available on the Web, give a good approach. He is a physician specialized in Chinese energy medicine, and demonstrates on various patients. His practical lessons are accompanied with explanations in English for the benefit of the students present at the demonstration. You can practice this massage on your own and already achieve an overall improvement of your circulation and the energy in your lower abdomen, including your sexual energy.

MASSAGING THE BELLY

The receiver is lying on their back on a massage table, or at least on a high bed. The lower body is naked to the waist: karsai nei tsang deals with the minor pelvis (belly and lower abdomen) and the inner faces of the thighs. There is no need for oil.

Standing close to the table, you move both hands in clockwise circles to distend the abdominal muscles and organs. Karsai compressions use three fingers. You dig them into points compressing the principal veins in the abdomen, and you maintain the pressure for some twenty seconds. Of the three central fingers, the strongest is the middle finger. Press on four levels, one after the other:
- below the ribs, right – middle – left
- in line with the navel, to the right and to the left of it.
- below the navel, in line with the dantian, our center of vital energy, right – middle – left
- just above the pubis, right – middle – left

These pressures activate the flow of blood back to the heart, which makes for a better irrigation of the genitals: either the penis and testicles, or the ovaries, uterus and vagina, as well as the essential organs (nei tsang in Chinese) i.e. the liver, kidneys, spleen, heart and lungs. You can also begin by pressing in the middle and then moving to the sides. The order is of no importance but your fingers must move downwards.

MASSAGING THE GENITALS

Once the receiver's circulation has been invigorated, move on to the genital area. Spread their thighs and fold their shins inward. Their ankles are at an angle such that the soles of their feet are face to face.

— Massage firmly the inner faces of the thighs and crotch on those "iron doors" which seal off the genital zone in someone who has a blockage. Your whole hand slides here with a little pressure, including the perineum and the bottom of the buttocks.

— Lay your fingers on the perineum, asking your subject to breathe several times through this point.

IF THE RECEIVER IS A WOMAN

— The massage is applied to the outside of the labia majora and the perineum with two or three fingers. The movements of your whole hand are directed towards the inner face of the thigh and the pubis by turns.

— Next you massage the inside of the labia majora using the yang touch, it is not a caress. You may knead-and-roll the labia majora between your fingers though this requires considerable dexterity for you mustn't pinch the very sensitive mucous membranes. At this point you may end the massage, or else go on to massage the labia minora if the receiver is willing to go further, as determined in your preliminary conversation. The labia minora are also massaged with the knead-and-roll technique or with a gentle sliding pinch along their whole length.

➤ Finish with your hand cupped over her genitals for a few moments.

IF THE RECEIVER IS A MAN

➤ Here, the massage of the penis and testicles is carried out with no ulterior intention. Use a firm, enveloping movement, with a little pressure (yang touch).

➤ Next you lay your fingers on the perineum and ask the receiver to breathe several times through this point. The perineum swells with inhalation and the fingers lying there press gently with the exhalation. Breathing in and out from 6 to 10 times is enough to bring more vital energy to that area which is already well relaxed and which is the object of the awareness and attention of both partners.

➤ If the receiver is sexually aroused, it is time to stop and restore the purely affective character of the massage by laying one hand over his heart, and cupping the other over his dantian.

The karsai nei tsang is not a form of foreplay.

THE KARSAI NEI TSANG SELF-MASSAGE TO RECHARGE YOUR BATTERIES

Duration: 5-10 minutes

POSITION: PRONE OR SEATED

➤ Begin by recharging your energy batteries using the method conceived by the Sino-Thai doctor Mantak Chia: rub your hands together to warm them, then apply both hands to the dantian beneath the navel and rotate them in small circles, scarcely moving them. Make some 80 rotations in one direction and 80 more in the other. This will warm your vital organs (nei tsang) by activating the blood circulation in this area.

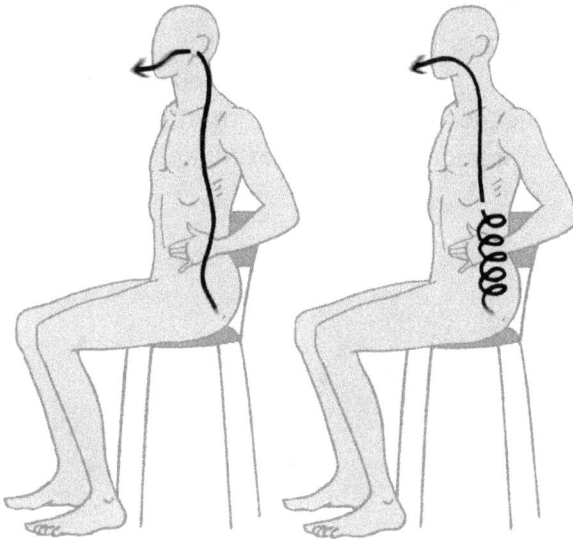

Figure 42. Vital organs self-massage.

— Next lay two or three fingers of each hand on either side of your navel. Press and release, accompanying this alternation with fairly quick breathing.
— Now press on your navel with three fingers, as in the karsai nei tsang massage and hold this position for 30 seconds, eyes closed, tongue lying against your palate with the tip touching your incisors in order to generate the electric current which will recharge you.

The warmth which you diffuse through the inside of your body will rid you of the chill which weakened your organs and glands. Smile and think of yourself as using the energy of the planet to recharge your batteries.

The Butterfly
Eliminate the emotional stress lodged in the iron doors (your crotch and the upper inner faces of your thighs) with a yoga position: sitting cross-legged, thighs apart with the soles of your feet pressed together, relax that part of your body.

Chapter 19

TANTRIC GROUP PRACTICES

WATSU, CRADLING IN WARM WATER

Duration: a full evening or all day Sunday

The watsu (*water shiatsu*) dates from the New Age years and is again back in fashion. Cradling is the main dish of a series of exercises and interactions carried out in a small, heated swimming pool under the supervision of a coach. Water restores our unity and possesses incomparable healing and soothing powers. Our breathing rhythm produces a gentle rocking. There is an undeniable connection between water and the origins of life. Sessions may be mixed or single-sex.

Requisites

- A towel, a bar of soap, shampoo and a beauty lotion to smear over your whole body during the shower which follows the session in the pool.
- Provisions for the convivial picnic afterwards.

Like in every Tantric exercise, each person is focused on his or herself. Ultimately the Other has no other function than that of a catalyst, triggering a state of consciousness and our awareness of our inner power.

The physiotherapy pool is lit with candles. Ten to twelve people get into the water. Our bodies are naked, light and weightless.

— We hold hands in a motionless circle long enough to be anchored to the pool floor and feel connected with the
— group. We take deep breaths, exhaling with our mouths open to get rid of any tension.
— Next we stimulate a reciprocal awakening of our energy points by connecting with ourselves, one hand on our own heart, the other on the sacrum of the person next to us, stimulating the energy lodged in the first chakra, the root chakra.

All the playful exercises that take place in the pool involve touching the other members of the group. Our encounters with the Other take place mainly through our sense of touch because we keep our eyes shut as much as possible.

After the awakening comes the cradling. One, two or three participants induce vibratory movements in the body of a person who is floating on their back, just beneath the surface of the water so that they feel submerged.

➤ One of the cradlers keeps the person's head above water by supporting the back of their neck. The body is sustained by one or two pairs of arms and gently rocked from side to side. After 10-15 minutes, the rocking subsides. The person is put back on their feet in the pool.

CRADLING FOR COUPLES ONLY, MIXED SESSIONS

The woman is often the driving force in a couple that takes the plunge: she is the one who wants to bring about a change for the better in the relationship and takes it on herself to convince her partner to come with her to a watsu evening. The coach's instructions will sometimes turn these sessions for couples into aquatic love coaching. But let there be no mistake about it: mixed evenings involving men and women who do not know each other, make no allowance for fantasy fulfillment despite the nudity of the participants. Groping hands and libidinous intentions are severely frowned upon! In a preliminary phone conversation, the coach can discourage anyone who hopes for another type of get-together, laying stress on its spiritual and playful dimensions. Participants are quickly immersed in a sensual and sensorial state of mind which goes far beyond sex.

The exercises enable us to better know ourselves, to liberate unused energy and strengthen our self-confidence. This type of interaction also helps restore our lost confidence in the Other, whom we can begin to view differently in a more spiritual intimacy. At first, some intimidated women keep their swimsuits. But generally they remove them in the course of the evening, when their fear of the gaze of the Other has worn off. The water and the rocking have a reassuring, maternal effect. When we go home again, we feel reconciled with all the parts of ourselves.

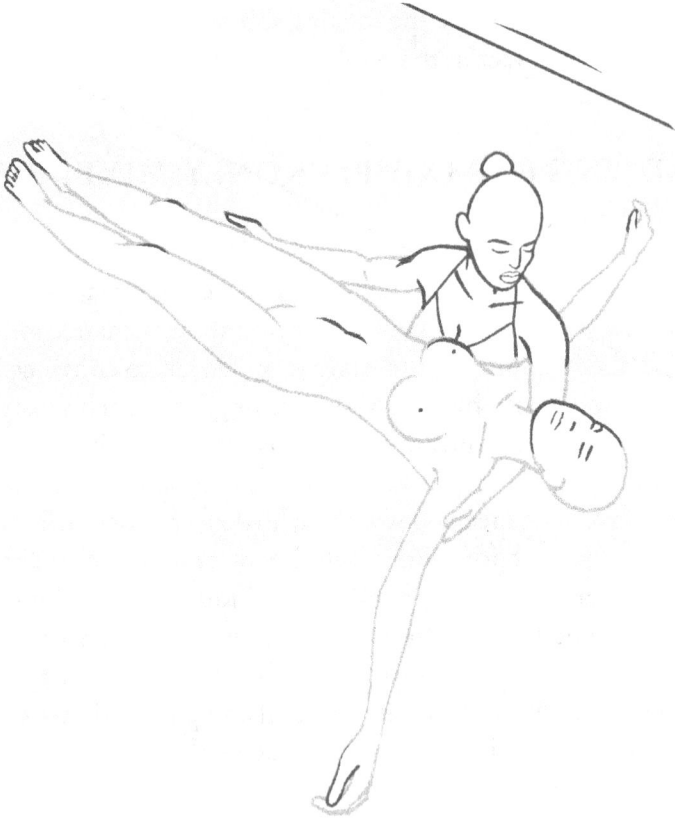

Figure 43. Watsu.

TANTRIC AND KASHMIRI MASSAGES

Watsu may also be carried out in the warm waters of the South Seas. With the development of the self-help fashion, the luxury and thalassotherapy resorts around the Caribbean and in Asia might well take it up for their clientele.

WATSU SESSIONS FOR WOMEN

Duration: 3 hours

This cradling in warm water produces powerful effects. We feel by turns mother and newborn infant, sometimes even a foetus in our mother's placenta. This is an effective way of becoming reconciled with womanliness, to place in perspective our relationship with our mother if our filial relations were bad. You emerge from these sessions calmed and joyful, in tune with yourself, energized and spiritually strengthened.

For some people, this rocking has a regressive effect. They are back in their mother's womb. Others drift off into a daydream. Others experience strong emotions, surges of affection. We discover ourselves in a state of nature, sometimes with the very first experience of cradling, when the layers of our humdrum existence, the cares and affects of everyday life have been stripped from our thoughts.

In another exercise, our thoughts focus on a positive theme, as in meditation. This may be tenderness, joy, love, peace, giving, beauty, sharing, etc. Interactions with the energy points of the different participants are associated with this meditation. These vibrations bring about a liberation of energy.

A sharing of food, nuts, dried fruit and cakes prolong this moment of pleasure and light spontaneity. We return home unburdened and happy.

WATSU SESSIONS FOR MEN

Duration: 3 hours to one day

Coaches supervise the male groups, generally on a Sunday or a weekday evening. These bring together men who are gay, bi, or straight, all interested in exploring their masculinity, the riches of manliness in heart, body and mind. A man who had a bad relationship with his father may find here a way of firming up his own identity. Men rarely have the opportunity of communing with other men without judging them or competing with them. Immersed in warm water, they mirror themselves in each other, stripped of their mask, bereft of their ego, in all simplicity. They listen to the needs of the Other, in silence. Fraternity, empathy, insouciance, the freedom of childhood revisited, affectionate, attentive men open their arms, cradle and love. They let themselves be guided, get in touch with their inner self and bind with other men. The emotions brought out by this sharing flow freely and shamelessly. Every man comes out stronger and in tune with himself. A man who had a bad relationship with his father may find here a way of firming up his own identity. The "men only" pool is a bubble of enveloping gentleness, a moment of confidence which gives rise to a feeling of mutual support and the sensation of rediscovering one's humanity. Needless to say, there is no sex-play in this group.

TANTRA TRAINING COURSE

Duration: a weekend

Requisites
- A Yoga mat or perhaps a cushion if one or the other is not provided
- One or two bath towels
- A pareo
- A bottle of water

Combined with the Tantra itself, the connection established with strangers commands our respect during the simplest Tantra course. We experience several emotional and sensual sharings with the group or with one other person. We mustn't lose sight of the fact that the heart is at the root of any Tantric practice: love illuminates each episode of sharing in the course of these exercises.

Our goals are letting-go, gaining confidence in ourself and the Other, allowing our emotions to surface and our personal development. Whether or not the Tantric massage is part of the program, a successful course will enable us to take charge of our mental activity and to win an empowerment impervious to the prejudices and dictates of society. Above all, we are committing ourselves to a personal quest for fulfillment. Later, experiencing several Tantric or Kashmiri massages will complete the opening of our hearts with specifically bodily feelings.

IN A COUPLE

When there is a decline of intimacy in a couple, taking part in a Tantra course (or a Tantric massage) will reawaken our capacity to experience emotions: the body is reconnected with the heart. We invent new caresses, new gestures, forms of thoughtfulness and surges of affection capable of reviving the pleasure of being with our usual partner. The innocence of these moments of sharing will resuscitate the teenage sensations we have forgotten.

For some of us, who have never experienced anything of the sort, it is an extraordinary discovery. It is possible to heal some of the wounds of life, sufferings we have repressed and which still lurk deep within us. Such a cure will bring to the surface new perceptions of our relationship with the other person: we will look differently on the body and on sex.

Workshop take aways

"You are perfect!" This is how the organizer of a Tantric workshop called "The Five Elements" greets us, the participants who have entered the big room after hanging up our coats and taking off our shoes. The Coué method of self-persuasion dies hard it seems, since if we are perfect then we need nothing. Shaking or the dance of Shiva dispels tension. Exercises with another person include eye-gazing and the sense of touch to connect with the Other. The atmosphere becomes less strained. We take pauses around a teapot where a Yogi tea is brewing: proverbs tied to the sachets offer conversation pieces during the respites. Nobody dances any more in nightclubs where you stand around chatting, glass in hand. Here, a bit of dancing around a herbal tea bar gives us a chance to move our bodies and do ourselves some good! In the end, the content of a Tantra session matters little; the important thing is to get to know yourself and subsequently other people through these group practices.

A TRAINING COURSE IN TANTRIC MASSAGE

Duration: a weekend
(or several weekends for a gradual initiation)

Requisites
- A bar of soap, shampoo
- An oil bottle, if it is not provided

Being on the receiving end of a Tantric massage is often a preamble meant to prompt us to learn the rudiments. You'd better have a massage with an experienced person before agreeing to go with them on their next training course: this will enable you to get to know their protocol and their style... or to look elsewhere if these don't suit you! Tantra massage is a potluck affair. There are plenty of interesting courses, and others that are best avoided. The choice of a person with whom you will feel at ease is of prime importance if you are to find fulfillment there.

Most courses involve equal numbers of male and female participants and are supervised by two coaches, a man and a woman, unless it is a single sex course. Several Tantra-linked exercises will precede the massage proper. First, we get into the mood. The Tandava dance (dance of Shiva) loosens our pelvis and limbs and connects us with cosmic energy. This is a meditation in movement in which you are your own partner. Exercises of eye contact or touching establish our connection with the other participants. We become conscious of our bodily limits in this intimate, silent confrontation with the Other. As we become more experienced we can push our exploration further. The alternative to dancing is shaking our whole body including our head for 10 minutes. This is guaranteed to relax us! (See **Chapter 2**).

Next we get down to cases. Self-massage first, then a micromassage with a partner of either sex. We focus on our movements, on the correct position relative to the recumbent body, on the handling of the oil-bottle. These are the things that will absorb all your attention as a beginner. The course will enable you to master the basics. Once you are familiar with a few good movements, you can devote yourself to your own perceptions, or refine them in your couple.

A TANTRIC MASSAGE WORKSHOP

Duration: an evening or a whole day

Requisites:
- A towel or pareo
- A pair of slippers or socks

Your hankering to try your hand at massage will materialize in a workshop, even if you don't commit yourself to a whole weekend. You won't master the art of massage after a single workshop session but you will have the precious opportunity to practice with different partners in roomy, pleasant surroundings. This way you can try different touches and learn from more experienced practitioners in order to improve your personal technique. Beginners are welcome. The participants are not all experts, masseurs and masseuses of various levels rub shoulders. You may well encounter professionals who come to share a moment of conviviality and freely practice their art.

The hall, studio or gym is laid out with mattresses or padded mats and bottles of oil.

- The workshop begins with a round of talking. Participants introduce themselves.
- We get to know one another by marching or dancing together, frequently changing partners for twosomes, etc. according to the coach's instructions.
- When it comes to the massage phase proper, we will try our hands at both roles, changing partners often. Sometimes we are blindfolded so as not to know whom we are massaging.

My advice
If you are a beginner, don't be afraid of being ridiculous or awkward. Others are no more advanced than you are. The conviviality of a workshop, experimenting physical contact with partners, understanding one another through your hands, will provide nourishment and help you to improve.

Chapter 20

TANTRIC SEXUAL TECHNIQUES

IN A COUPLE

Complicity and openness will enable each partner to contemplate the rediscovery of their body and that of their lover thanks to Tantric massage. This will be a wonderful discovery for a couple trapped in a routine. This type of massage helps us to see and feel differently, more completely, from the top of our skull to the tips of our toes, to become aware of ourselves by re-appropriating our own body and playing on our partner's body as we would play on a musical instrument.

Who will be the first to give? Which one of you will lie down and receive? If your partner is tired, become the giver and prefer the traditional free-style Tantric massage, with long sliding movements. Ask your partner to lie face down. Start by massaging their back, not their genitals. When the receiver turns over, the second part of your massage becomes more sensuous. At this stage, you are on your knees between the receiver's feet. Move between their thighs to massage their breasts or pectoral muscles, then their belly. The massage may possibly be followed by intercourse. The receiver is under no obligation to reciprocate by giving you a massage the same day.

GENITAL ANATOMY

THE PERINEUM (PC MUSCLES)

Located between the pubis and the coccyx, the perineum muscles serve to arouse us, whichever gender is considered and whichever form of sex is chosen. The perineum is at the base of the abdomen and supports, among other organs, the anus and the genitals. The contractions of the pubococcygeus (PC) muscles in that area enable us to achieve our own arousal and liberate some of the sexual energy stored at the base of the sacrum. If these muscles are in trim, it will keep our genital organs young as well as our urinary function: by building them up, we retain our urine, which is essential to avoid little urinary leaks as we grow older. If we are going to exercise only one single set of muscles in our body, this is it!

The *Jen Mo* point as the Chinese call it, often referred to in the context of acupuncture and acupressure, is located at the center of the perineum. The left side of the anus corresponds to the left side of the perineum and the left kidney, the right side to the right kidney and the liver. Contracting your PC muscles to keep them toned up can be done anywhere and at any time. Female Tantrikas keep them toned with stone eggs (carved in amethyst, pink quartz, etc.) keeping these *Ben Wa* balls in their vagina while going about their usual business. Some fortify them after giving birth by carrying a pair of *Ben Wa* balls for several hours a day. Men increase their control over their ejaculation with specific exercises. (See below the exercise "bolting the door" in the section dealing with men).

Anus and rectum

The rectum, the end of the digestive system for defecation and excretion, is composed of a first section positioned towards the navel and lined with muscles meant to prevent incontinence, and a second section inclined towards the spine. Both these sections are full of nerve-endings and muscles with sphincteral functions. The first or anal section can be contracted at will when we tighten our anus.

IF YOUR PARTNER IS A WOMAN

THE FEMALE GENITALS

VULVA

The labia majora extend from the pubis —called mons veneris— to a point some 2 or 3 centimeters from the anus. They surround and protect the labia minora —also called the nymphae— the clitoris, the urinary meatus and the mouth of the vagina. They are sometimes hairy on the outside, sometimes naturally hairless, and very often plucked. They are sensitive to the kneading-rolling technique but also to being pinched when closed, which compresses the labia minora and the clitoris and excites a woman enormously. When she is aroused, they swell and become moist with a natural liquid secreted by the Bartholin's glands located at the back of the vulva.

Clitoris

The equivalent in the female of a miniature penis is the culmination of a woman's pleasure. In order to see a clitoris with a short tip protruding from the rear of the vulva, one must pull apart the labia majora. A remnant of the primal undifferentiated sexes long before birth, it consists of a Y-shaped spongy mass whose branches extend 8 or 10 centimeters beneath the pelvis and whose tip surrounds the urethra and the mouth of the vagina. This tip thus surrounds the urinary meatus and swells up at the entrance to the vagina forming two bulbs called the vestibular bulbs, the "vestibule" being the little pink hollow at the mouth of the vagina. It has a sort of cowl, corresponding to the foreskin on the penis, while the erectile section corresponds to the male glans.

Like the penis, the size of the clitoris varies from one woman to another. It can be so long that it sticks out between the labia majora like a little tongue, or, on the contrary, tiny when at rest, lying discreetly in its niche. What you see of it, nestling between the labia majora and the urinary meatus, is only the tip of the iceberg, the part that rises and swells in the event of sexual arousal. Compared with the vagina, which has few nerve-endings, the only function of this appendage is to convey to the brain the pleasurable sensations it feels when caressed by a finger or a tongue. The clitoris contains over 8,000 nerve-endings, as against 4,000 in a penis. Well vascularized, it swells up and triggers the lubrication and opening of the vagina entrance. This appendage's cowling, called the glans, is the outer part, some three to five millimeters long. It is connected to four roots 10-15 centimeters long, surrounding the vagina.

The clitoris plays an important role in the female orgasm, but it may provide only limited pleasure when it is the only part of the body stimulated. A Tantric massage does not dwell on it.

Labia minora

These are an extension of the clitoris and surround the entrance to the vagina. Their size is proportionate to the clitoral glans and in some women may extend beyond the labia majora. They swell up along with the clitoris and are also lubricated from within by the Bartholin's glands.

Vagina

Moist and elastic, the entrance is about five centimeters in diameter, and is surrounded by tiny labia. It leads to a tunnel of mucous membranes some 10 centimeters long, capable of dilating to make room for a newborn child... or a large penis. During foreplay, glands secrete lubrication. There are only two to three centimeters of nerve-endings on the walls of the vagina.

THE RENOWNED G -SPOT

It is located on the front wall of the vagina. It can be felt with the finger. It is the size of a small coin and its texture differs from that of the rest of the vagina. It is convex, grainy and fleshy. It is a remnant of what will become the prostate gland in a male child, a spongy excitable body. A short penis or a finger can stimulate it, generating intense arousal.

The stimulation of the G-spot may trigger multiple orgasms, but also, in some women, a female ejaculation which is a prelude to orgasm, a mixture of prostatic phosphatase and glucose. Female ejaculation is quite common after fifty.

THE A-SPOT

This is also located on the front wall of the vagina, a third of the way from the neck of the cervix. This is another tiny, very smooth, spongy mass. It is a sensitive area in the event of deep penetration.

THE VAGINA BOTTOM

Located at the back of the vagina, this is an orgasmic zone at the entrance to the cervix, stimulated by deep probing in a woman who appreciates this type of penetration. The rest of the vagina has no nerve-endings. In the absence of any foreplay involving the clitoris and the G-spot, the vagina will not be lubricated and will remain insensitive.

SOLO FEMALE PRACTICES

SELF-MASSAGE OF YOUR BREASTS AND VULVA

- Sit with bare feet on the floor or a sofa folding one leg so that the heel is pressing against your vulva. Keep a steady pressure on that spot. If you're not flexible enough, sit on a rubber ball. Practice circular breathing and don't forget that inner smile.
- Warm your hands by rubbing them together. Lay your palms over your breasts and feel the warmth entering them. Slowly massage your breasts in small inward circles. Do the same in the other direction. Alternate this massage with light applications of pressure on your sternum. Use your mind to direct the energy drawn from your breasts towards your genitals, remembering to circulate it throughout your body by your breathwork: it must irrigate all your glands including your ovaries.
- Lick your lips while you massage yourself, thereby stimulating another gland, your pancreas. The compassionate energy brought forth by massaging your breasts will rid you of the negative energy accumulated in your liver or spleen, it will charge them with positive energy.
- Next place your hands on your knees and feel the energy from your breasts coursing through your body. With each breath, send it in thought to your ovaries. Move your labia majora and minora on the ball or your heel. Now you are ready for an internal orgasm.

PRACTICES IN A COUPLE

STIMULATING A WOMAN'S SEXUAL ENERGY MASSAGING HER BREASTS

Duration: 10 minutes

The woman is lying on her back on a mat while the man is kneeling or seated on the floor behind her head. This massage may be carried out with or without gel. The hands move in circles, broad movements at first, becoming increasingly tight. Both hands stay in contact with the woman's breasts at all times. This massage releases emotions, generates tenderness and ignites the fires of desire.

If a woman has her breasts massaged, it is not to be aroused, it is to re-appropriate a part of her body which is all too often neglected by her partner(s). And the same holds for our genitals, rarely fondled since the hygienic attentions paid to them in our infancy.

OM: ORGASMIC MASSAGE

Duration: 15 minutes

Requisites
- An exercise mat
- A bath sheet or large towel
- A few cushions
- Lubricating gel

Because her sex-life was inadequate, confined to the perfunctory foreplay of her partner followed by penetration, an American woman named Nicole Daedone felt estranged from her companion and no longer wanted to make love. With an eye to having stronger sensations again, she invented a connecting technique based on a repeated massage of her clitoris by her partner. She calls this "orgasmic meditation" or OM. This clitoral massage enables a woman to concentrate on her own sensations because of her immobility: she does not have to move her pelvis as she would during intercourse. The idea is to free the woman of the need to give pleasure and focus on her own. Her partner has to concentrate on the woman's genitals to which he normally pays only passing attention.

You create a comfy nest on the floor with a large towel and several cushions. The woman removes her skirt or slacks and her panties. She keeps the top to forestall any irrelevant temptations: the man might become aroused, which would spoil his massaging, introducing a particular intention. She lies back comfortably with her head on a cushion. Her partner sits by the right side of his companion's pelvis (if he is left-handed he sits on her left and the following indications must be reversed). He places a cushion under her left leg at knee-level, straddles her thighs and her right leg and lays her other leg on his own thigh.

The woman may if she wishes hold the man's ankle to create a contact. She keeps her eyes shut the whole time. Unless he turns towards her, the man does not see his partner's face. He may look at her vulva and clitoris to make sure what he is doing with his finger.

— Now sir, you begin by caressing the inside of your partner's thighs.
— Apply a gob of gel on her clitoris and begin by putting the thumb of one hand next to the mouth of the vagina, the middle finger of the other hand at the upper end of the vulva.

> After a few motionless seconds, move your finger down to the clitoris. Move up and down, up and down...
>
> The lubricant will create a sort of cushion between your partner's clitoris and your finger. Repeat this stroke slowly for 15 minutes.

After the massage, each partner will describe to the other their impressions and sensations. It may be that both will remember a moment when they felt bound by a strong tie, a common sensation.

STIMULATION OF THE G-SPOT AND THE VAGINA

> Insert one lubricated finger into your partner's vagina. Keep it there for at least twenty seconds without moving. Energy rises in the vagina, the uterus, and the ovaries and spreads through the abdomen to the heart. If you feel tensions, gently massage the area by sliding your finger along the vagina wall. Lay another finger on the forward tip of the clitoris, towards the pubis. Withdraw, then start again.
>
> Insert a second finger into the vagina. Study the person's reaction when you move your fingers and proceed intuitively. Stroke, press, pause for a few second to diffuse the energy, then resume.

> Press on the G-spot, a surface the size of a walnut located at the front of the vagina from one to four centimeters from the vulva according to the individual. The size of the point will vary as well, just as different men have different sized penises. Hook your forefinger or your index finger for a gentle caress. Press the G-spot with your fingertip, then release. Do it again gently. Twist your wrist while you massage the vagina up and down but without going in all the way. Move in and out several times being attentive to your partner's reactions.

If the vagina opens and grows moist, it is an invitation to go further. If the woman you are massaging moves her pelvis in a way which invites you to insert your fingers further, do so and twist your wrist some more.

— If your partner is very aroused and her vagina is wide open, insert a third finger. Caress the vagina, twisting your wrist. Half way into the vagina, you stop. Remain motionless for several seconds. Withdraw a little. Then move in again slowly. Repeat the same cycle: pause — withdrawal — advance, and keep twisting your wrist.

— Spread the sexual energy evenly through her whole body by caressing the insides of her thighs, buttocks and belly, either after you have withdrawn your fingers or with the other hand. Your hands should often remain motionless for periods of 10 seconds.

IF YOUR PARTNER IS A MAN

THE MALE GENITALS

PENIS

This is the organ for erotic games and intercourse. It is composed of two cavernous bodies and one spongy body surrounding the urethra and the glans. The foreskin covering these forms a mobile cowling over the glans called prepuce, which religious Jews excise 8 days after birth in a rite called brit milah, but this is also the case with most US males for reasons of hygiene, since the folded skin can be a place of incubation for germs if it is not regularly washed. The two faces of the prepuce are separated by a ring of skin. Its inner face is a mucous membrane and its outer face protects the emerging glans in the event of an erection. At the center of the glans lies the urinary meatus, the open end of the urethra, which runs through the center of the spongy part and channels the flow of urine.

Testicles

These two egg-shaped gonads hang in the scrotum and become looser with age. The testicles have two purposes: reproduction of the species thanks to the spermatozoa contained in the sperm, and the secretion of male hormones. They swell up when the male subject is aroused.

Prostate gland

Located just over the bladder, it serves to produce the seminal liquid in which the spermatozoa are immersed and which nourishes them. This gland measures several centimeters in diameter, is protected by a sort of capsule and surrounds the base of the urethra.

The equivalent of the woman's G-spot is called the P point and is located on the rear wall of the rectum, two or three centimeters from the anus. A massage of the prostate via the anus (rectal exam, sodomy) can arouse a man to the point of ejaculation. The pleasure of sodomy is due to the fact that both sections of the rectum are full of nerve-endings and muscles with sphincteral functions and also that the very excitable prostate is located just behind the intestinal wall. Massaging the prostate is sometimes included in a Tantric massage. (See below at Prostate massage).

SOLO MALE PRACTICES

TESTICLES MASSAGE

To tone up your own sexual energy, warm your palms by rubbing them together. Take your testicles in your right hand, keeping your left hand on your pubis (or the other way around if you are left-handed). Massage your testicles in little circles, always in the same direction. Chinese Taoists recommend massaging them 81 times! Rub your hands together again. Repeat the massage in the opposite direction.

THE LOCK-DOWN EXERCISE

This exercise enables a man to control the rise of his sperm. Standing in the horse position, pull your chin into your chest. Alternatively you may sit on the edge of a chair, feet flat on the floor and spread to shoulder-width. The tip of your tongue is pressed against your palate, just behind the front teeth.

➤ Now masturbate, and when you are very aroused, inhale deeply through the nose while clenching your fists and jaws as tightly as you can and keeping your tongue pressed to your palate, your feet clenched like two claws sucking in the space above the floor, pulling on your buttocks, abdomen, pelvic region and anus. Maintain this contraction so as to keep your sperm inside you.

➤ Now let go all at once and the body will relax. Energy flows into your genitals. At the end of the exercise, send the energy down to your navel, where your vital energy is stored.

The purpose of this exercise is to gain complete control over your genitals, the ultimate goal, which is hard to achieve, being to have orgasm without ejaculating. The Taoists recommend contracting the lower abdomen muscles 9 times in succession while taking a deep breath through the nose.

Precautions to take:

- Do this exercise on an empty stomach
- Don't breathe through the mouth
- If you tend to exaggerate everything you do, be careful: sexual energy is very powerful and might overwhelm you to a degree that it would be hard to control
- Don't expect spectacular results the first few days
- Be careful if you have high blood pressure
- This exercise is not suitable for men with prostate problems

EXERCICES FOR TWO

BRINGING OUT THE ENERGY IN A MAN'S GENI-TALS

Duration: 10-15 minutes

The object of this massage is not to give him a hard-on but to tame the penis of man who is not always self-confident. You can get rid of the anger and frustration which might be lodged there. This form of touch also has a healing effect on the person doing it. Whether the man has an erection or not is of no importance.

➤ Begin by running a confident hand over your partner's genitals. Do it again several times until you feel that area of his body has relaxed. The touch of your hand should give your partner confidence in a climate of love and dispel any unconscious fears.

➤ With your closed fist, massage the first chakra, located between the rectum and the penis, with a series of pressures on the Jen Mo point, located at the center of the perineum. Little by little, you will press harder. If you have some degree of intimacy with your partner (which is probably the case as this type of massage is intimate) move on to a massage of the penis, but this must not be a caress. It is important to stop before the orgasm and ejaculation, of course. Avoid moving up and down on the shaft: that will trigger his ejaculation, which is not the goal of a Tantric massage.

➤ Massage the testicles by taking them lightly in your hand with a slow rotation (yang touch). Remove you hand frequently from your partner's penis to spread the energy to the inside of his thighs and his belly in order to integrate.

Slip the edge of your hand between his buttocks, and massage with two or three fingers the rim of his anus where anger and frustration are lodged. Finish with a laying on of hands, one cupped over the penis, the other over the heart.

PROSTATE MASSAGE

Duration: 15-30 minutes

This is a therapeutic massage meant for men who have a hard time holding back their ejaculation, and those who have erection problems following a prostate operation. It reveals the sensual dimension of this organ.

Preparation

The receiver will have followed a meatless diet for two days and given himself an enema the day before so as to have a clean anus and rectum when it is time for this massage. The rectum requires artificial lubrication to be penetrated. The mucous membranes are fragile and the person giving the massage must wear a rubber glove.

Requisites
- Rubber gloves
- A lubricating gel

The receiver is lying on his back. The giver strokes (yin touch) and massages (yang touch), first the perineum between the base of the scrotum and the anus, then the anus itself with the pads of their finger. The anus will contract as soon as it is touched and so you must mollify it. The gloved and lubricated active finger must be pointing towards the belly in order to follow the curve of the rectum. The middle finger is best suited for this. Once it has softened the entrance to the rectum with very small movements, it will encounter a firm excrescence: this is the prostate. The feeling produced by your finger pressing on the P point is unusual, it is both pleasant and unpleasant.

— When the receiver becomes accustomed to this, the giver inserts a second finger or a third and presses lightly on the prostate. You may choose to massage by pressing or by making tiny circles with two or three fingers (yang touch) or simply running your fingertips lightly over the mucous membranes (yin touch).

Massaging the prostate by an insertion of fingers, a penis or a dildo (rectal examination, sodomy) may arouse the man or trigger an ejaculation.

Repeated therapeutic massages of the prostate will enable a man to discover the sensual dimension of that gland and can help heal problems of premature ejaculation. It is in any man's interest to develop his PC muscles (see Solo Tantric stimulation) in order to control his ejaculation. With a little practice he can achieve multiple orgasms.

Diffuse sexual energy

A man's sensibility is one hundred times greater during a genital massage than during masturbation. Between two specific caresses, don't forget to diffuse the sexual energy generated to his belly, torso and buttocks with ampler caresses throughout the massage: this is the integration phase. Breathe deeply, and pay close attention to the breathwork of the both of you.

CONCLUSION

Like tango dance-steps, these protocols and these techniques are merely crutches to help you begin. Give your imagination a free hand to stimulate your creativity: you're a free agent! After you've tried a few massages, your hands will be guided by your sensibility and as you gain self-confidence you will derive full enjoyment from these moments of sharing. But don't forget to open your heart. That is the basis of the Tantra. Be in close touch with your partner, heart to heart, during the preliminary ritual, but during the laying on of hands as well. Your sensibility and your love are transmitted through your hands.

Whichever massage you choose, Kashmiri, karsai, Tantric, energetic, emotional, etc., giving the same type of massage several times will help you get to know yourself better, and will open you up to the happiness which comes with an awareness of the present moment.

www.ingramcontent.com/pod-product-compliance
Lightning Source LLC
Chambersburg PA
CBHW060847280326

41934CB00007B/954